Menopause

Jill Wright MNIMH

D0755058

HERBAL HEALTH

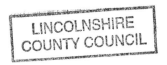
Published in 2001 by
How To Books Ltd, 3 Newtec Place,
Magdalen Road, Oxford OX4 1RE, United Kingdom
Tel: (01865) 793806   Fax: (01865) 248780
email: info@howtobooks.co.uk
www.howtobooks.co.uk

British Library Cataloguing in Publication Data
A catalogue record for this book is available from
the British Library

Edited by Diana Brueton
Cover design by Shireen Nathoo Design, London
Produced for How To Books by Deer Park Productions
Designed and typeset by Shireen Nathoo Design, London
Printed and bound in Great Britain
by Bell & Bain Ltd., Glasgow

Note: The material contained in this book is set out in good
faith for general guidance and no liability can be accepted for
loss or expense incurred as a result of relying in particular
circumstances on statements made in the book. The laws and
regulations are complex and liable to change, and readers
should check the current position with the relevant authorities
before making personal arrangements.

Herbal Health *is an imprint of*
How To Books

Contents

8 Case histories

List of illustrations

Preface

Are you feeling hotter on occasions than you used to? Do you wake up sweating at night? Does your heart suddenly thump for no reason or feel as though it's missed a beat? If your periods are lighter, or more irregular, if you can't shed weight as you used to and you suffer from vaginal soreness, if you are over 40 you may be starting the change of hormonal status which leads to **menopause**.

It is common now to talk about the **peri-menopause**, which includes all the years in which you are still having periods, but experiencing the symptoms mentioned above which indicate changing hormone levels. Some women complain of mood changes such as irritability, emotional lability, and loss of libido (interest in sex), but these are not definitely linked to hormone change. Most of the symptoms mentioned so far can also be caused by stress and anxiety, so this book will give help in differentiating stress related symptoms from hormonal ones.

Most women find that periods have stopped altogether by the age of 55 and many women arrive at this point (true menopause) without any of the symptoms mentioned above.

We are now warned of the hidden body changes which happen at this time, such as reduction in bone density and rise in blood cholesterol levels. Most doctors suggest that all women take medical treatment, such as **Hormone Replacement Therapy** (HRT), for these conditions.

- You may have tried HRT and found it didn't agree with you, causing water retention, digestive disturbance or unwanted mood changes.

- Perhaps you have a history which prevents you from considering HRT – a hormone–dependent cancer, or a family history of such cancers, or maybe you have an increased tendency to thrombosis.

- You may prefer to maintain your mid-life health without using medication, for ecological, sociological or ideological reasons, or because of concerns about unknown long-term effects of HRT.

- You may simply not wish to continue a monthly physiological cycle indefinitely, or have doubts about the efficacy of synthetic hormones.

These are all reasons why you might need an alternative to HRT. Herbal medicine is the leading alternative to orthodox drugs and there is new, exciting research into **plant hormones** which reveals how herbs and vegetables can play a part in maintaining our health through menopause.

As a member of the National Institute of Medical Herbalists for ten years, I have treated a great number of women with menopausal problems in my clinic. In retail practice, I have answered countless queries and given general advice on how to deal with hormonal imbalances. In this book I have written down the answers to the most frequently asked questions. I offer practical advice on how to treat these conditions, when to consult your doctor and how orthodox as well as herbal medicines work. By reading this book you can find out how you can:

- Use herbs to eliminate hot flushes and palpitations
- Improve your emotional balance
- Settle menstrual irregularities
- Increase absorption of nutrients
- Improve energy and overall health.

You can also:

- Learn how to make simple herbal remedies and combine herbs to suit your individual needs.

- Understand labels on over-the-counter remedies, information in leaflets and pre-operation advice.

- Get more from visits to doctors, hospital consultants and alternative therapists.

A brief guide to the processes which happen in the female body will make you feel more confident in discussing your health with professionals.

The advice contained in this book is meant to be for general use only. If you have a specific medical condition or an allergy, or are taking medication which may affect your use of herbal medicine, you should consult a qualified health care professional such as a doctor or a medical herbalist before starting to use herbal remedies at home.

Jill Wright

❧ 1 ❧

Understanding
the menopause

All about the female reproductive system

There are two aspects of the female reproductive system:

- the **organs of reproduction**
- and the **hormones** regulating the processes which take place within them.

There is also a command centre for reproductive hormones situated in two connected nerve centres in the brain. These are the **hypothalamus** and the **pituitary**.

The Hypothalamus and the Pituitary

These nerve centres secrete hormone-like substances which travel to other areas via the blood stream.

- The hypothalamus secretes **releasing factors** which cause the pituitary (also known as the hypophysis) to secrete **stimulating factors.**

- These in turn stimulate the production of **hormones** and other secretions in the target organs (ovaries, womb, vagina, breasts) and movement in accessory organs (fallopian tubes, cervix, vagina).

- The hypothalmus and pituitary also control **thyroid hormone**, **growth hormone** and **adrenal hormones**.

- One part of the hypothalamus (linked to the pineal gland) responds to changes in levels of light which tells us when to sleep and when to wake up.

- It also affects the **releasing factors (tropins)** which in turn regulate pituitary hormones, so that they are produced in 'pulses' at different times of day.

- This effect is carried on all the way down the hormone 'tree' (see Figure 1) so that all hormones are produced in varying amounts during the 24-hour cycle. These are called **diurnal rhythms**.

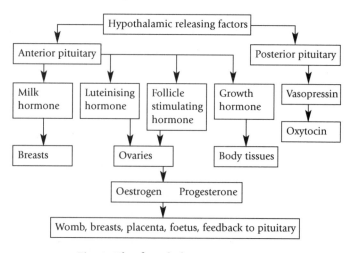

Fig. 1. The female hormone system.

It is important to remember that the hormones produced in the hypothalamus and pituitary centre, which affect reproductive organs and sexual development, are part of a larger **endocrine system** which includes the **thyroid**, **pancreas** and **adrenal gland**. Another fact of interest is that females also make male hormones (and vice-versa). This may result in imbalances which herbal treatment can help.

Hormone functions

Hormones act on cells all around the body to increase or decrease their activity. This affects all vital processes in the body, especially growth and reproduction, but also the speed at which our body processes run – known as metabolic rate. Hormones travel in the blood stream, and can be measured there by taking samples for analysis.

Hormones
Growth Hormone

Growth hormone enables the body to undergo changes as we age, such as developing longer bones, more muscles and fat in areas characteristic for our sex. Growth hormone:

- Increases protein-synthesis, giving greater muscle mass, dense bone and cartilage and decreases starch use for energy
- Increases use of fats for energy and hormone synthesis

- Is secreted throughout life, under special control during pregnancy
- Responds to protein deficiency in starvation and to other hormone changes.

Prolactin (milk hormone)

Prolactin is produced in especially large quantities in pregnancy but is also produced in regular quantities at other times in a woman's life. Excessive prolactin production is commonly recorded in pre-menopausal women and causes pre-menstrual problems. It:

- Increases the number of milk glands in the breast (leading to temporary growth in size)
- Stimulates milk production, under special control during and after pregnancy.

Follicle stimulating hormone (gonadotropin 1)

Follicle stimulating hormone ensures the normal process of egg development and release in the ovaries, as well as contributing to the balance of ovarian hormones. It:

- Causes growth of the sac around each egg in the ovaries
- Increases secretion of oestrogen in ovary tissue.

Luteinising hormone (gonadotropin 2)

Luteinising hormone contributes to the balance of ovarian hormones, and ensures the normal process of ovulation as well as preparing the womb for pregnancy. It:

- Adds to the stimulus of oestrogen production in the ovaries

- Makes follicles rupture, allowing egg release (ovulation)
- Adds to the stimulus of progesterone secretion in the ovaries.

Oxytocin

Oxytocin is a hormone produced by pregnant women during and after birth. It affects the chemical balance of womb muscle, ensuring normal delivery and expulsion of the afterbirth, as well as aiding breastfeeding. It:

- Makes womb muscle contract to deliver a baby
- Causes milk glands to contract and expel milk.

Oestrogen (oestradiol and related compounds)

Oestrogen is the most well-known of the female hormones, with a large number of effects in the body. It is responsible for the overall female shape, and building adequate tissues to support pregnancy. It affects women's health in many ways, particularly by its actions in the blood circulatory system. It:

- Stimulates the growth of fat, muscle, bone and hair cells during puberty
- Stops bones lengthening at 16 years
- Stimulates the growth of tissues lining the womb (endometrium) in a cycle
- Increases mucus secretion and maintains the lining of the vagina
- Increases sebum secretion of skin
- Possibly maintains libido (not proven)

- Aids salt and water retention
- Increases blood clotting
- Causes nausea in pregnancy.

Progesterone

Progesterone is often thought of as the hormonal balance to oestrogen. It:

- Supports the breasts and womb for healthy foetal development and feeding
- Increases the growth of glands in the womb lining and breasts
- Controls muscle contraction of the womb, preventing miscarriage and enabling the expulsion of unwanted womb-lining at menstruation
- Thickens mucus and maintains linings of the vagina
- Raises metabolic rate.

The monthly cycle

Oestrogen and progesterone act together to create the monthly female hormone cycle. Oestrogen and progesterone are both produced in the ovaries, which contain thousands of follicles (immature egg sacs). Oestrogen is secreted by the tissues of these follicles when they are stimulated by hormones from the pituitary – follicle stimulating hormone (FSH, gonadotropin 1).

When the follicle is halfway through its cycle of growth, the extra oestrogen it is producing stimulates (by feedback) the production of luteinising hormone (LH, gonadotropin 2). This makes the follicle grow bigger and faster, increasing oestrogen production until it 'bursts' and releases an egg (ovulation). The remainder of the follicle tissues (now called the **corpus luteum**) then secrete progesterone, with smaller amounts of oestrogen. About two weeks later menstruation occurs.

Male hormones in the female body

Follicle cells in the ovaries also produce hormones called **androgens** such as **testosterone**. These are precursors for female hormones and are converted to oestrogens both in the ovaries and also in fatty tissues all over the body. This fatty tissue is an important source of oestrogens for the woman after menopause. Androgens are also produced in the adrenal glands. They are responsible for male patterns of sebaceous gland, bone and hair growth. If they are not metabolised into oestrogens in the female, they can cause male type characteristics such as acne, facial and body hair. Androgen production is increased by extra adrenal activity such as under severe stress, very vigorous frequent exercise or starvation.

Day 1	Lots of FSH / Some LH / Lots of oestrogen
Day 10	Sudden increase of FSH and LH
Day 12	Ovulation
Day 14	Lots of progesterone / more oestrogen / less FSH
Day 28	Low oestrogen and progesterone

Fig. 2 The monthly female hormone cycle.

How the body maintains a balance of hormones

Hormone balance is usually achieved by feedback mechanisms (see Figure 3). **Positive feedback** describes the process which happens when there isn't enough of a hormone. Messages are sent from receptors to the pituitary and then to the hypothalamus causing an increased production of releasing and stimulating factors. **Negative feedback** consists of messages telling the control centre that there is sufficient of a given hormone, so that production is slowed down.

Prolactin, oestrogen and progesterone are all part of a complex feedback system which is also affected by factors such as nervous tension, exercise levels and diet. When the system doesn't function properly, excesses occur which cause menstrual problems and hormonal imbalance syndromes.

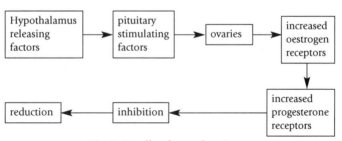

Fig.3 Feedback mechanisms.

The menopause explained

Strictly speaking, menopause is the end of menstruation, when the last follicle matures and releases its egg.

Changes in menopause:

- Fewer follicles remaining in ovaries
- Reduced response in ovaries
- Fewer hormones from hypothalamus and pituitary
- Less oestrogen and progesterone
- Skin and hair changes
- Mood changes.

The hormonal changes which occur in the female body take place over a long period, often as long as ten years between 45 and 55. It is now common to call this time the **peri-menopause** as it is obvious that the monthly cycle is still taking place while the events of change go on.

Peri-menopause

Gradually the number of follicles diminishes so that the ovary makes a smaller response to hormones released from the pituitary. This leads by feedback to fewer hormones being released from both hypothalamus and pituitary.

Periods may still occur, because eggs are still being released, but the overall level of hormones is smaller, so that there may be:

- a thinner lining to the womb (less oestrogen)
- less mucus and lubricant lining to the vagina (less progesterone).

These two changes lead to:

- lighter periods
- and vaginal soreness or dryness.

Other reasons for menopausal symptoms

Skin and hair changes are not directly related to hormone status, as age is the main factor here. Men undergo much the same changes –drier skin, thinner, wirier hair, less bum!

Some women experience more frequent periods. This is not well understood but is due to changes in feedback to the pituitary and may also be a feature of thyroid dysfunction or stress.

Many women also experience very heavy periods and prolonged bleeding at this time. This is more often due to development of **fibroids** – benign outgrowths from the womb wall. These are usually age-related but are not necessarily a condition associated with menopause. In fact they frequently stop causing problems when periods cease, as the hormones which make them proliferate are no longer produced in sufficient quantities. Occasionally an imbalance of hormones is the cause of excessive bleeding from the womb. You should consult with a doctor about excessive bleeding, and eliminate any more serious disorder before you start a course of herbal treatment.

Loss of sex drive (libido) and emotional irritability are often associated with the menopause, but there is no definite evidence that the female hormones are responsible for maintaining sexual interest or for producing calmer feelings.

Why do some women have an earlier menopause?

Most of the variation between individual women is down to genes in the same way that balding in men depends on their genetic inheritance. There has been no link established between the age of menopause and the age at which women start menstruating. There also appears to be no link between menopausal age and number of children women have. However there are some factors which do affect the onset of menopause, such as diet, work and exercise. Surveys show that women in the 'first world' affluent countries generally have later menopause than in 'third world' poorer countries.

Stress and menopausal symptoms

The hypothalamus is also responsible for regulating temperature, circulation and sleep rhythms, so disturbances in feedback to this nerve centre cause irregularities in:

- temperature control – hot flushes
- sleep patterns – early waking
- and circulation – palpitations.

It is wise to remember that stress, anxiety and adrenal responses have identical effects, as well as causing mood changes. It is therefore very important to note if stressful times are associated with more menopausal symptoms, or if periods of relaxation bring about a reduction of symptoms. It is common to find that women experience almost complete relief of symptoms while on holiday.

It is also worthwhile remembering that women between 45 and 55 generally have teenage children, elderly parents, demanding jobs, loving husbands and lived-in houses. These are enough to place a strain on the most saintly personality. For the average woman, the general stress of life reaches its maximum in the peri-menopausal years. Many women begin to build up levels of anxiety at this time which are detrimental to health and enjoyment of life. As mentioned before, anxiety and depression can affect hormone balance, which makes the physical changes of menopause problematic.

Hormonal	**Other Causes**	**Stress-related**
Osteroporosis	Fatigue	Migraines
Dry skin	Heavy period	Depression
Vaginal atrophy	Frequent periods	Loss of libido
Weight gain		Irritability
High cholesterol		
Hot flushes		
Palpitations		

Fig 4. Changes in menopause.

How anxiety affects your hormones

Stress and illness are registered in the brain, which activates various parts of the nervous system, getting you ready for the famous 'fight or flight' response. All glandular activity is slowed down and adrenal activity stepped up. You may not be able to actually fight or run, so this 'energy' may be diverted into other reactions, such as anxiety, irritability or depression. The adrenal hormones cause dilation of blood vessels in muscles, constriction in skin (hands feel cold), increased heart rate, dry mouth, less digestive secretions and a sense of mental and physical tension.

These symptoms are very similar to those caused by rapid hormonal changes. If the stress is repeated you can suffer chronic stress adaptation symptoms, ie long-term hormone imbalances. This is a very good age to reassess your life, look at what you want out of life and consider making changes.

Osteoporosis

Many doctors now recommend that all women take HRT to protect their bones from osteoporosis. This is a condition in which the bones become brittle and break easily, causing distress and pain to some women as well as real danger by complications to elderly women.

Osteoporosis occurs more readily in women because oestrogens inhibit the breakdown of bone. In fact they prevent bone making cells from being converted into bone destroying cells. This is still a controversial area of medicine, because there is insufficient research into the 50% of women who do not suffer loss of bone density, or into the mechanism by which men suffer (or don't suffer) osteoporosis and the evidence for HRT treatment of osteoporosis is still being gathered. There has been a huge rise in the number of osteoporotic bone fractures in women over 50 since the 1960s, so there must be other factors affecting women's health to account for this change.

Recent research has suggested that the number of times a woman ovulates in her lifetime affects the likelihood of her developing osteoporosis, so that prolonged use of the contraceptive pill, which suppresses ovulation may be linked with the onset of osteoporosis at or before menopause. Operations which remove the ovaries would have the same effect, as well as extreme physical exercise and eating disorders such as anorexia. These are all known factors which may contribute to the change in patterns of female bone health and more research is needed to establish their degree of importance.

2

What conventional medicine can offer

Most women who visit their doctor with menopausal symptoms will be offered hormone replacement therapy – HRT. There is a growing trend of recommending HRT to all women over 45 as a protective (prophylactic) against osteoporosis and high cholesterol, whether they have risk factors for these or not. Risk factors are:

- Family history of the same disorder
- Dietary factors such as high-fat, low-fibre diet
- Lifestyle factors, such as smoking or immobility.

Hormone replacement therapy (HRT)

HRT consists of oestrogen and progesterone replacement, using **natural oestrogens** derived from horse urine, and progestogens:

- oestradiol
- oestrone
- oestriol.

Conjugated oestrogens is the term given to a combination of natural oestrogens. There are **synthetic oestrogens** available, these are:

- ethinyloestradiol
- mestranol
- diethylstilboestrol.

Progesterons includes:

- progesterone
- didrogesterone
- hydroxyprogesterone
- medroxyprogesterone
- norgestrel and derivatives.

Progestogens are normally prescribed with oestrogens as a tablet to be taken in the second half of the monthly cycle, because oestrogens cause the womb-lining to over-thicken if taken on their own and this carries a high risk of cancer. These hormones are supplied in much larger amounts than the body's natural (endogenous) production, to offset losses through digestion and tissue dispersal.

How HRT works

HRT preparations replace endogenous (a woman's own) hormones. They act on peripheral tissues (target cells) in the same way as described on page 18, but they send negative feedback to the hypothalamus, which reduces the production of releasing and stimulating factors. Side effects occur because they are given in higher doses than endogenous hormones and they disrupt the fine-tuning of the positive and negative feedback processes.

HRT brands

The main brands of HRT (oestrogen and progestogen combination) are:

- Premique
- Climagest
- Cyclo-progynova
- Elleste.

These consist of separate tablets which are taken at different times in the monthly cycle to mimic the normal increase in progesterone in the second half of the cycle. The quantities of oestrogen contained vary by up to 100% between brands of tablets.

Patches

Patches are a type of plaster applied to the skin and which contain female hormones. They are more uniform, releasing much smaller amounts of oestrogens over a longer period. These don't pass through the digestive system, so this method is closer to the body's natural production of hormones. However progestogen has to be prescribed in tablet form to accompany oestrogen patches. Common brand names are:

- Estrapak
- Femapak
- Evorel.

Each pack contains two types of patch, one for each half of the cycle, and the pack also contains progesterone tablets.

Post-hysterectomy

Women who have had their womb removed (hysterectomy) can also choose from a range of oestrogen-only preparations, both patches and tablets. Brand names include:

- Climaval
- Elleste-solo
- Estraderm
- Fematrix
- Menorest
- Progynova.

Gels and creams

Some gel agents such as Oestrogel and Sandrena are available. Women who use hormone gels are advised to avoid skin contact with males, as the systemic absorption is high. There doesn't appear to be any precise advice as to how much skin contact to avoid!

Oestrogen creams such as Ovestan for local treatment of vaginal atrophy are available, but these are also highly absorbable and women are advised not to use them for more than six weeks, and in phases of two to three days at a time. Some creams also destroy latex in condoms and diaphragms, so alternative contraceptive methods have to be used.

Advantages and disadvantages of HRT

There are many research trials which show that women who take HRT have better bone density than women who don't, but the trials generally don't look at lifestyle, ethnic and dietary factors when comparing women. Research does show that being thin, European or Asian, smoking and drinking a lot of alcohol increase a woman's likelihood (risk factor) of suffering from osteoporosis. There doesn't appear to be any information on exercise and dietary effects on risk factors. To gain this protective effect, HRT is recommended for peri-menopause and several years beyond menopause. Some experts suggest that 15 years is optimum for effect.

This advice conflicts with evidence that the risk for breast cancer increases slightly for every year a woman takes HRT.

The risk for thrombosis (clots blocking a blood vessel) is also increased by taking HRT because exogenous (medicinal) oestrogen increases clot formation. It is possible that diet and exercise may offset this risk, but unfortunately there is no research into this type of 'combination therapy'.

Oestrogen-only therapy protects the heart and lowers

cholesterol, which may help to avoid gallstones but progestogens greatly reduce this protective effect. Oestrogen-only therapy clearly increases the risk of womb cancer, even when applied as a cream vaginally.

There doesn't appear to be any evidence that HRT helps insomnia, although it is frequently suggested that it might.

Who should and should not take HRT?

To summarise, women who have a family history of breast or womb cancer, or of thrombosis and women who have varicose veins or are obese should be advised *not* to take HRT.

The Committee on Safety of Medicines recommends that women without these risk factors should take HRT for a short time around menopause to help to avoid what they describe as a small increased risk of breast cancer, associated with longer term use of HRT. They feel that the benefits of HRT outweigh the risks. Women with a diagnosis of osteoporosis should consider using HRT as a therapeutic agent, unless other factors prevent it.

Unfortunately, heavy smokers and drinkers also have risk factors for heart and circulatory disorders as well as cancer. Menopause could be a good time for them to change their habits, so that more options are open to them with less associated risks.

The Side-effects of HRT

Many women complain about annoying side-effects of HRT, which they often say are worse than the symptoms of menopause. Water retention, weight gain, breast tenderness and bloating head the list, with migraine, indigestion, nausea, constipation and fibroid problems following close behind. These effects result from the larger dose of hormones entering the body all at once, or in amounts which upset the balance achieved by the natural feedback systems.

Concerns about these effects and what many women see as medication without a cause, make women look for alternatives. This is the subject of the next chapter.

Treatments for osteoporosis

Biophosphonates are prescribed for osteoporosis. They work by sticking to bone and preventing it from breaking down. Brand names are:

- Didronel
- Fosamax
- Bonefos
- Skelid.

These are drugs which often cause severe irritation to the gullet, so great care has to be taken in managing them. They also interfere with mineral metabolism all over the body, so can have a lot of serious side-effects. They are saved for severe cases and, used with caution, can reverse osteoporosis.

Raloxifene is an oestrogen-derived compound which improves bone-density but increases clotting, so has to be taken with an anti-clotting agent.

Treatments for anxiety and depression

Many women consult their doctor for anxiety and depression which they asssociate with the menopause. They are generally prescribed anti-depressants. In the past the same age-group would have received tranquillisers. The most widely-used are Amitryptilene and Imipramine (MAOIs) and the SSRIs – Prozac family, Fluoxetine, Paroxetine and Seroxat.

MAOIs

These act by preventing the destruction of chemicals in the brain such as noradrenaline. This helps to make you more relaxed and lifts the mood.

What are the side-effects?

They also affect other systems which use this chemical transmitter so cause a dry mouth, blurred vision and urine retention. There are worries that long-term use (more than six months) of these drugs destroys the body's own ability to do this job, so that intractable depression sets in when patients try to cease taking them.

SSRIs

These act by preventing the re-uptake of a chemical transmittor called serotonin, so that it remains in the circulation and a feeling of relaxed confidence pervades.

What are the side-effects?

These are usually temporary, but can be severe. The main problems are headaches, nausea, loss of appetite and insomnia. These usually subside after two to three weeks but insomnia sometimes persists for longer. There are reports that long-term use (more than six months) produces a sort of 'euphoric despair' which may result in destructive or inappropriate behaviour. There are even cases of suicidal tendencies.

It should be suggested that all anti-depressant use is accompanied by some sort of 'talking therapy' so that real causes of anxiety and depression are not missed. If you are considering using this group of drugs, you should make firm plans with your doctor for time-limits to treatment, and plans for what to do when you cease taking them. This is yet another reason to look at the menopause as an opportunity to review, assess, evaluate and change!

Sleeping pills

The pattern of prescribing these has changed, mainly for
political rather than medical reasons. In the 1980s, when
doctors became obliged to account for the cost of their
prescriptions, many began to question the validity of long-
term prescriptions for sleeping pills – often continued for
20 years or more. The main types of sleeping pills used
nowadays are called benzodiazepines – brand names are:

- Nirazepam (also called Mogadon)
- Temazepam
- Flurazepam
- Diazepam.

How do they work?

They enhance a neurotransmitter called GABA, which is
involved in controlling messages from the brain for
movement. This chemical reduces brain activity and so
helps sleep.

What problems do they cause?

Despite assurances from the manufacturers and the
Medicines Safety Committee, these sleeping pills make it
more difficult to fully wake up in the morning. This is
known as the hangover effect and results from the drug
not having been completely eliminated from the body.
This is a variable effect, which depends on the individual's
constitution and balance. Some people complain of not

being 'focused' until mid-morning when they take benzodiazepines at night. They are well known for causing the paradoxical effect of irritability and anxiety, especially in long-term use, because of interference with other brain neuro-transmitters.

The effects of ceasing these pills are noticeable, with increased and more intractable insomnia, anxiety, sweating and tinnitus (ringing in the ears). It is best to reduce doses gradually by cutting into halves, then quarters over a few weeks.

Treatments for itchy skin

Skin becomes drier with age and this can cause itching. Generally topical treatments are used, although sometimes mild sedatives have been tried, such as those contained in anti-histamine tablets. The preparations available to your doctor fall into four main groups. They are all intended to reduce itching by adding moisture to the skin and soothing nerve endings.

Group 1 Petrochemicals – liquid paraffin and wax

Includes:

- Aqueous cream
- Emulsifying ointment
- Alcoderm
- Diprobase
- Unguentum.
- Drapolene
- Epaderm
- Ultrabase
- Vaseline

Group 2 Petrochemicals and lanolin

Includes:

- E45
- Hewlett's cream
- Kamillosan
- Keri.

Group 3 Peanut oil

Includes:

- Hydromol
- Oilatum.

Group 4 Contain urea in a petrochemical, lanolin or vegetable base

Includes:

- Calmurid
- Nutraplus.
- Balneum (made with soya oil)

Problems with these preparations

All the creams made with petrochemicals are very greasy. Many herbalists believe that greasy creams block the skin's pores and cause heat to be retained, making most skin problems worse. Petrochemicals can also cause the skin to become drier in the long-term and may upset the natural bacterial population (flora) which helps to protect the skin from infection.

More research is needed to compare emollients (soothing preparations) of plant, animal and petrochemical origin. Many women are sensitive to lanolin (woolfat), which can cause irritation and redness, whilst others are allergic to nuts, or may work with children who are hyper-sensitive to nuts. Vegans and vegetarians prefer not to use animal products, ecologists may prefer to rely on renewable sources of oils. Details on how to make your own creams are given in Chapter 5.

Treatments for vaginal dryness and soreness

This condition includes vaginal atrophy, where tissues lining the vagina are thinned. Topical applications consist of:

- **oestrogen creams** – Orthodinoestrol, Orthogynest (both contain peanut oil)
- **oestrogen pessaries** – Tampovagan
- **oestrogen rings** – Estring.

You must take progestogen tablets if these are used for more than one month, as oestrogen on its own can cause overgrowth of the womb lining which may lead to cancer. The 'minimum effective amount' is recommended by doctors, but it is obviously difficult to monitor the amount used and quantities of oestrogen vary a lot between brands. The instructions for use vary as well so that it may take some time to find the right dose and judge the effect.

One disadvantage of topical applications for the vagina is that they may damage latex condoms and diaphragms (Orthogynest and Orthodinoestrol are noted for this). As pregnancy is still possible as long as periods are occurring and even up to one year after the last period, this is a fact worth noting.

A final note on the cost of HRT

Currently the average cost of a monthly supply of HRT pills is £6, and of patches £10. This is paid partly by the NHS where there is a difference between the cost of the drugs and the price of a prescription. In Hertfordshire alone there are 110,000 women aged between 45 and 64. If they all received a subsidy of £2 per month on their HRT, it would cost the NHS well over two million pounds a year. Multiply this figure by the number of counties in Britain to obtain a huge sum of money being spent on medication which is not necessary for many women.

Some doctors argue that it is cheaper to treat the menopause than osteoporosis (which costs £34 per month, on average) and associated fractures. This is true on an individual basis, but over half the women receiving HRT do not have osteoporosis, so it might be a lot cheaper for all of us, and with no medical risks, to use scans to establish who has bone density problems and needs treatment. It would be even cheaper to find out why osteoporosis has increased since the 1960s and prevent it from happening. Statistics and medical records show that tuberculosis was almost eradicated from Britain, not through innoculation, but through improvements in diet and living standards. The same might be true of osteoporosis.

This book hasn't been written to win an argument on the benefits and costs of HRT but to present the facts and alternatives. A large number of women don't want to take orthodox hormonal therapies during the menopause years. They are worried about side-effects, inconvenience and long-term effects. In the next chapter we will look at the alternatives and find out if they really work.

3

Using herbs to treat menopausal problems

Herbal medicine is the leading alternative to orthodox pharmaceutical treatment. When herbalists make up a prescription for women in peri-menopause they take into account all the factors which contribute to her health and try to improve all the systems which are affected by hormonal changes. This is called a wholistic approach. It is the main difference between conventional treatment and herbal treatment. In addition to prescribing herbal medicine, herbalists would want a patient to start exercises and dietary changes in a strategy to maintain general well-being, including bone and heart health.

Aims of herbal treatment

- Improve digestion
- Balance hormones
- Reduce nervous tension
- Improve circulation
- Support overall health.

We use herbs which improve digestion and circulation, increase elimination of water via lymph and kidneys, relax mind and muscles, improve liver function and balance hormones.

There are many herbs which have a unique action on the female hormone system. Some contain ingredients known as **phyto-oestrogens** and **isoflavones**. Others are believed to have a **progesteronic** action, although ideas about these actions are changing all the time. There is increasing evidence for their effectiveness but little knowledge about how the herbal hormones work. There are several modes of action which are outlined in the section on hormonal agents (page 52).

How herbs work

Herbal constituents

Herbs contain small quantities of chemicals compared to modern pharmaceutical products, which extract or synthesise one chemical in much larger amounts to obtain an effect. Most herbs contain a large number of active constituents which work together to create one or more effects. The more we find out about herbs, the more we realise that each constituent is a valued part of the whole. Negative effects are balanced by positive ones.

St John's Wort

A good example of the balance within many herbs is

found in St John's Wort. Recently much has been made of a research trial which showed that a St John's Wort preparation made liver enzymes more active, which reduced the effect of other drugs taken at the time. Although this trial didn't examine women taking the oral contraceptive pill, it was assumed that this effect would extend to it. The St John's Wort preparation used in this trial was standardised to contain a larger amount of one constituent – hypericin – than all the others. Not only has hypericin failed to show anti-depressant activity on its own, in repeated trials, but another constituent – hyperforin – has been shown to counterbalance hypericin in its effect on liver enzymes. Many other research trials on St John's Wort have shown no adverse effect on drugs taken simultaneously and doctors in Germany continue to prescribe it as a relaxing anti-depressant.

In Britain doctors are advised to warn their patients that their oral contraception may not be safe if they take St John's Wort and herbalists caution patients to use non-standardised forms of this herb in moderate quantities if they are taking medication with a 'narrow therapeutic range' (where small alterations in dose make big differences in effect). There is no direct evidence that St John's Wort affects the contraceptive pill and no reported cases of pregnancy while combining them, but NIMH members would advise patients who are worried about this to use extra contraceptive methods or change to another herbal remedy.

Synergistic chemicals

Similar bad publicity surrounds liquorice, where a constituent called glycyrrhizin is thought to raise blood pressure, but in fact dozens of other constituents act to lower it, in particular by diuresis (elimination of water).

- Where two or more constituents act together to create the same effect, this is known as **synergy**.

Some herbs, like garlic, contain several ingredients which provide help for our circulation on multiple levels. Its antibiotics protect against infection and repair the damage caused by wear and tear on the insides of our blood vessels. Digestive stimulants help the absorption of sugars and fats from the bloodstream. As a circulatory tonic it reduces the stickiness of platelets, dilates the capillaries, causes mild sweating and increases kidney activity, and so helps to protect against strokes, lowers blood pressure and helps to protect the heart from strain in exercise.

- This type of multiple activity is a feature of many herbs which enable them to support the wholistic approach very well.

How long do herbs take to work?

Although some herbs act swiftly, like the sleep-inducer Valerian, herbal remedies generally act slowly and their effects are cumulative. They gently rebalance physiological processes as though switch after switch is thrown until the full effect is achieved. This can take weeks, sometimes months, but it is worth waiting for as the risk of side effects is very low, due to the tiny amounts of chemicals involved.

Valerian appears to improve the quality of your sleep as well as helping you to doze off and it doesn't cause a sluggish feeling in the morning because the chemicals contained in it are in small amounts and are cleared from the body fairly quickly. This lower level of activity may be disappointing if you want to be knocked out, but using herbs like Valerian as part of a plan to restore sleep patterns can be effective.

How do herbal remedies get to their target?

Herbal compounds need to be absorbed across the wall of the digestive tract, so they have to be released from their structures – stem, root, leaf, flower or berry etc. – first of all. Hot water and alcohol do some of this job for us, so that teas and tinctures are more easily absorbed than tablets and capsules, which need to be broken down physically before the active chemicals are separated from the inert matter to which they are attached. All food and medicine passes through the liver (in the blood circulation) before it finally enters the body tissues, where it is used.

Sometimes, chemical compounds need help in crossing through the wall of the digestive tract into the blood stream. **Carrier chemicals** can be attached to compounds

and ferry them through channels in the gut lining.
Hydrochloride is frequently found to be part of
conventional drug names as it has this function.

Do herbs have any advantages over modern drugs?

Herbal compounds often have an advantage over
synthesised chemicals in this respect, that they have
naturally occurring carrier chemicals already attached to
them. This is what is meant by **affinity**. Herbs are said to
have a greater affinity for the human body, like spare parts
dedicated to a particular engine made by the same
manufacturer.

Are herbs safe?

All the herbs which British Herbalists use are safe when
used in the correct dose for the right ailment. The herbs
mentioned in this book have been selected for their safety
in untrained hands, although you may need professional
help with your diagnosis. The National Institute of
Medical Herbalists (NIMH) maintains an extensive data
bank and works with government watchbodies to ensure
safety of its herbs. Recently some attention was given to
the group of compounds called pyrrolizidine alkaloids,
present in several plants, including comfrey, because they
can cause (reversible) damage to the liver if ingested in
large quantities. The evidence on comfrey is not based on
human case studies and the research involved feeding rats
exclusively on large amounts of comfrey. There is only

one reported case of human toxicity world-wide, which concerned a woman who took comfrey tea many times a day concurrently with illegal drugs in high doses over a long period. Several governments, including that of Britain, made moves to ban its use. After extensive discussions with the NIMH it was agreed to limit use to the guidelines given above, and restrict the root (which contains more P.A.s) to external use only. In this way herbalists acknowledge the potential risk and demonstrate the history of safe use.

Whole plant preparations stand the test of time

Although there are variations between plants around the world, herbalists believe that plants would only have gained a historical reputation for certain effects if their constituents were robust enough to maintain the same effect wherever they were grown or whatever minor differences there might be between local plant populations. Rosemary is distinctively Rosemary whether it's grown on a London balcony or in a Caribbean back yard. If only one variety in one particular year made someone feel better, its reputation would not have stood the test of time. The current trend, based on scientific research, is to standardise the process of growing, harvesting and storing herbs, so that their use is sustainable and patients get the best value from them.

Medical herbalists also recommend using whole, unaltered preparations, so that each constituent is represented in natural amounts. This is the type of preparation on which traditional knowledge is based and which you will be able to make at home. Don't forget that smell and taste are still very reliable indicators of the effectiveness of herbal medicine. It is also useful to remember that people vary much more than plants do!

Combining herbs with orthodox medication

Some drugs are altered by liver enzymes, so that they enter the main blood circulation in a different form. Some herbs (especially bitter tonics) stimulate the liver cells to work harder, or cause more liver cells to be active and this can affect other drugs because the liver removes them from circulation before they have had a chance to do their work. Digoxin is one of these and it is also a drug with a 'narrow therapeutic window'. This means that the difference between an insufficient, a beneficial and a harmful dose is very small, so that small changes in the amount getting through to the blood stream may result in the drug not working as it should. Two other drugs like this are Cyclosporin, used to prevent transplant rejection, and Phenytoin, an anti-epileptic. It is very important to check with a qualified herbalist and let your doctor know if you are adding herbal medicine to medication you are currently using.

There are many herbs which can be taken safely with other medicines, so don't feel deterred from trying, but do seek professional advice. Herbs can be used to offset the side-effects of necessary medication, like indigestion or nausea. They may enable you to take less of a remedy which you need, but which has troublesome side-effects. The important thing is how you feel, and that you don't endanger your health. It may be simple to ask your doctor to monitor blood levels of drugs and adjust the dose if necessary.

It would not be wise to embark on herbal medicine without medical supervision if you are on anti-psychotic medication, as you may not be aware that your mental condition has deteriorated when your current medication ceases to work. You may have strong feelings about the disadvantages of your drugs, but may not realise how your behaviour is changing and affecting others badly. It is possible to have herbal medicine for other complaints while on medication for psychosis.

Drugs to be careful with

- Anti-arrhythmics
- Anti- epileptics
- Anti-psychotics
- Immune suppressants
- Anti-cancer drugs.

Conditions to be careful with

- Pregnancy
- Epilepsy
- Schizophrenia, psychosis
- Organ transplants
- Allergies.

Herbal applications

Herbal applications for menopause include:

- Relaxants
- Hormonal agents
- Digestive stimulants
- Bitter tonics
- Circulatory tonics.

Relaxants

Herbal relaxants relieve tension and restore nervous activity to a normal level, whereas sedatives reduce brain activity to below normal functioning level. The former can improve concentration rather than impairing it, so it is a good example of a balancing action for which herbs are well-known. These herbs work in two ways.

- Nervine relaxants act centrally, by reducing the brain's sensitivity to nerve messages from the periphery (skin, joints, muscles etc).

- Muscle relaxants act peripherally, on nerve centres in the spinal chord, or on nerve endings in the skin, reducing the number of messages sent from the periphery to the brain.

Nervine relaxants tend to act centrally, muscle relaxants act peripherally, many herbs do both at once.

Hormonal agents

There is a large group of herbs providing chemicals which have a hormonal effect in the body. The most well-known are **phyto-oestrogens**, but there are also herbs with **progesteronic**, **testosteronic** and **adrenal** actions. These have a number of modes of action.

- Some block the actions of human hormones by occupying their sites in target organs. This may account for the known protective actions against hormone dependent cancers.

- Some may do the opposite and create more receptors for a hormone in a target organ.

- Some give feedback to the pituitary and hypothalamus to alter the production of hormones.

- Others provide building blocks (precursors) to make hormones, or act directly like hormones by occupying receptors and having the same hormonal effects.

Some herbs, like Wild Yam, have been used for the extraction of hormonal drugs used in conventional medicine.

There is unfortunately very little research into the way individual herbs act. In many cases we can only assume their action by the effects they have. We group herbs into:

- oestrogenic
- progesteronic
- and adrenal

types, according to their effects. For example Sage reduces the frequency and severity of hot flushes, so we assign it to the oestrogenic group, as we assume that the falling oestrogen levels at menopause account for this symptom. In fact the picture is more complicated, because many 'flushing' women show normal levels of oestrogen, whereas some who have low oestrogen experience no hot flushes. We must assume either that receptors for hormones are diminishing, or the feedback mechanism is failing, or some other factor is at work (or home!).

Digestive stimulants

Digestive stimulants can be used to increase the secretion of the digestive organs by stimulating **enzyme** action in the liver, as mentioned before, or by increasing the production and flow of **bile** (the bitters are noted for this action). Spices such as Cayenne, Ginger, Horseradish and

Mustard act by irritating the secretory linings of the stomach and intestines, causing increase in all sorts of secretions including **mucin**, which protects the stomach from acid. These spices also cause dilation of blood vessels serving the gut wall, which helps to increase the absorption of nutrients. It is thought that pancreatic hormones may also be produced in response to some of these digestive herbs, so sugar, fat and protein digestion may be enhanced. This is the action we call digestive **stimulation**. It may increase the absorption and metabolism (breakdown and use) of the nutrients needed for good bone formation.

Bitter tonics

These tonics are unique to herbal medicine. Nearly every country has a national favourite, the French drink Gentian wine, Italians prefer Vermouth, Mexicans use Angostura and the British put their bitters in stouts and beers. You can still buy a formula known as Swedish Bitters from pharmacies. Aromatic bitter herbs are also found in cookery traditions all over the world. In Britain Sage, Rosemary and Thyme are used to improve the digestibility of meat and bean dishes.

How bitter tonics work

- Taste buds detect bitters
- Nerve messages are sent to the brain
- Reflex messages are sent to organs

- Liver, pancreas and salivary glands are stimulated
- Better absorption and elimination results.

Bitter taste buds are located at the back of your tongue. They are designed to detect poisons and trigger a gag reflex, so you spit out food which is bad for you. Humans can overcome the bitter revulsion reflex by three methods; telling ourselves it's good for us, adding nice flavours or adding alcohol! The body however, still working to the primeval instruction handbook, initiates a process to rid the body of unwanted chemicals. The liver produces more enzyme and bile in response to messages sent to the brain from the tastebuds. Saliva flows abundantly to cleanse the mouth, activity in the stomach and pancreas increases, resulting in better absorption of nutrients and elimination of toxins. Pre-dinner drinks are good for you after all!

Circulatory tonics

These relax and dilate blood vessels, which lowers pressure. They increase blood flow to all parts of the body including internal organs, lower cholesterol, improve the elasticity of blood vessels and make them less fragile as well as reducing clotting or platelet aggregation, so help to prevent thrombosis. Menopausal women often avoid using the herbs which stimulate blood flow (such as Chilli, Ginger, Mustard and Horseradish) because they also increase sweating, which can be intolerable for women who experience severe hot flushes.

Iron-rich herbs may be considered as circulatory tonics as they provide the essential mineral for formation and function of red blood cells.

The role of relaxation and exercise

The Wholistic Approach to Relaxation

Herbal remedies	Exercise	Hobbies
Relaxing herbs	Yoga	Crafts
	Gardening	Clubs
	Walking	Gardening
	Cycling	Reading
	Dancing	Music

Relaxing is an important part of improving health in middle age, because stress reactions can increased blood pressure and the cardiovascular symptoms of menopause such as hot flushes and palpitations. Herbal nervines can help to reduce stress, but should be used as part of a general plan to reduce the negative aspects of menopause. This should include dietary changes, which are discussed in Chapter 6.

Exercise

Exercise is important to relieve symptoms of stress, because it helps to use up adrenalin, which causes blood vessel constriction and sometimes aching muscles. It:

- Relaxes mind and muscles, so helps to regulate cramps during menstruation
- Increases blood flow to the limbs, which helps to protect against arthritis and rheumatism
- Reduces excess weight gain.

Exercise has another important effect which is very beneficial to women. It increases the activity of **osteoblasts** – the bone-making cells – so is vital for protection against osteoporosis. Some say that 'impact' exercise – running, skipping and hopping – is particularly important as the impact of the body against the ground causes effects in joints, such as an increase in synovial fluid secretion. Muscular exercise including brisk walking and cycling, also causes an increase in osteoblast activity, so bones are strengthened. Some sports physicians argue that high impact sports and exercise – jogging, ballet, squash, badminton – cause more wear and tear in joints than beneficial effects. Probably the benefit lies in moderate exercise such as walking, cycling and dancing! Carrying heavy loads also causes excessive wear and tear, especially on knees, so shopping trolleys should become trendy!

Yoga is particularly good for relaxing muscles and improving the range of movement in stiff joints. It is a system of exercises which developed over more than 1,000 years in India. Hatha yoga is the name given to exercise designed to help physical health. You can go to evening classes or get books and videos from the library. Work through the exercises slowly, increasing the range of movement each day. You can omit the more 'spiritual' aspects if they don't appeal, although they can be used to aid relaxation which is another major benefit of yoga.

Recently a piece of research showed that gardening is the ideal form of exercise for shifting fat! According to researchers slow, sustained exercise uses fat for energy, whereas short bursts of aerobic exercises are fuelled by carbohydrate first, so that blood sugar is depleted and hunger sets in quicker. Working in an allotment or vegetable garden gives relaxation, exercise, fresh air, good food and company, then you can go home to brew or preserve your produce!

How exercise helps in menopause

- Uses adrenalin
- Stretches muscles
- Increases blood flow
- Increases bone density
- Relieves stiff joints
- Reduces excess weight.

Hobbies

Outside interests are a very important way of relaxing, as they enable one to forget daily worries in concentrating on the task in hand. Crafts such as sewing and knitting have become unfashionable amongst work-oriented women, but they are surprisingly relaxing. Gardening, brewing, winemaking, painting and other handicrafts including model-making have been some of the activities which patients say 'save them from insanity!' Reading is more relaxing than TV watching, and music can change your mood very quickly. Joining interest groups and clubs can give you a new lease of life. Every local library now has a computer listing of the associations in your area, you are sure to find something to suit you. Evening classes can give you new skills which lead you in different directions, and they are astonishingly cheap. Menopause is a good time to try something new, so go for it!

4

Directory of useful herbs

You will need to use a number of strategies to relieve menopausal symptoms and improve your health. You can use the information in this section to select the right herbs. Dietary approaches are covered in Chapter 6. The case histories in Chapter 7 guide you in building classic recipes, or tailoring one to your own individual needs.

Herbs are usually categorised by their **actions**, each herb will have some **primary** and some **secondary** actions. In some the actions are of equal importance. To treat menopausal problems we use hormonal agents, circulatory tonics, iron tonics, relaxants and digestive stimulants. When you read the case histories in Chapter 7 you will see how this directory can be used to pick herbs from the various categories to suit your individual needs. You can choose from:

- Hormonal agents
- Circulatory tonics
- Iron tonics
- Relaxants
- Digestive tonics.

HORMONAL AGENTS

Anemone	Hops	Squaw vine
Beth root	Motherwort	White deadnettle
Black cohosh	Red clover	Wild yam
Chasteberry	Sage	
False unicorn root	Shepherd's purse	

Anemone

Latin name	Anemone pulsatilla
Origin	Europe, Asia
Part used	Leaf and flower
Dose	$1/2$ teaspoon to 1 cup
	Tincture 1ml, 3 times daily
Constituents	Volatile oil, saponins, tannins, resin, camphor
Primary actions	Relaxant nervine
	Anti-spasmodic
Secondary actions	Hormonal agent
	Alterative (see below)
How it works	Saponins are often related in structure to hormones. In anemone they are also stimulant to the liver, increasing bile flow, so help to improve metabolism of nutrients, especially fats. This action may help to protect against the development of gallstones, and the hormonal saponins affect both male and female hormone structure, though the mechanism is not understood. The volatile oil and tannins may be

responsible for the alterative action. This is an old term used to describe herbs which relieve both viral and bacterial infections. The nearest modern equivalent is an antibiotic, but antibiotics only act on bacteria, whereas the herbal compounds appear to increase the body's resistance to a variety of organisms. It was once considered a specific cure for measles. Its main use today is for nervous exhaustion, pain and inflammation in the reproductive system, especially in menopause. It is observed to stimulate secretion of all mucus membranes, and this may account for its use as a remedy for vaginal dryness.

Caution	The fresh plant should not be used as the oil is irritating to skin and mucus membranes.
Growing guide	From bulbs in a well drained, sunny spot.

Beth Root

Latin name	Trillium pendulum
Origin	North America
Part used	Root
Dose	1/2 teaspoon to 1 cup
	Tincture 2ml, 2-3 times daily
Constituents	Volatile oils, tannins, saponins, glycosides
Primary actions	Hormonal agent
	Uterine tonic
Secondary actions	Astringent
	Antiseptic

How it works   Beth root is a corrupted form of birthroot. This American settler name gives some idea of its use in helping to check haemorrhagic bleeding after giving birth. Tannins coagulate protein, including blood cells and bacteria, so aid clotting and reduce sepsis. They aren't absorbed from the gut so these chemicals can only be active on tissues with which they come into direct contact, such as the bowel wall and vaginal area if used as a douche. This action accounts for its traditional use in treating nose bleeds and thrush (where it halts fungal growth). It is likely that the saponins, together with the glycosides, have a hormonal effect on the lining of the womb, as they are related in structure to steroidal hormones. Beth root reduces the proliferation of endometrial (womb) tissue in the first half of the cycle, so we assign it to the progesteronic group, although we don't know exactly how it works to reduce blood loss during menstruation and after birth.

Growing guide   Prefers rich, damp, semi-shaded woodland soil. Low growing perennial.

Black cohosh

Latin name	Cimicifuga racemosa
Origin	North America
Part used	Rhizome
Dose	1/2 teaspoon per cup

	Tincture 2ml, 2-3 times daily
Constituents	Glycosides, bitters, isoflavones, volatile oil tannins
Primary actions	Hormonal agent
Secondary actions	Anti-spasmodic
	Anti-inflammatory
	Circulatory tonic
How it works	It has traditionally been used by Native Americans for female complaints. Its isoflavones bind to oestrogen receptors in the body, so have some oestrogenic effects, and the same chemicals are anti-spasmodic, helping to relax blood vessels, lower blood pressure and slow pulse rate. These actions also reduce the severity of palpitations. Its bitters help to remove sugars and fats from the bloodstream, which adds to the circulatory tonic effect. Some research has shown that black cohosh has been used successfully in conjunction with drug treatment for breast cancer. It appeared to reduce the severity of hot flushes and reduce the proliferation of breast tissue. This is what herbalists call a balancing action but it is not fully understood. It is very likely that other so called oestrogenic herbs will have the same anti-cancer effects, but more research into how they interact with drugs is needed before we can recommend them for use during chemotherapy. To be on the safe side we

recommend using herbs after chemotherapy is finished, as drugs like Tamoxifen still offer the best outcome for breast cancer sufferers.

Growing guide Tolerates semi-shade and prefers damp soil. Used to be popular Victorian garden plant, tall white spires of flowers, 4ft high perennial.

Chasteberry

Latin name	Vitex agnus castus
Origin	Europe, Asia
Part used	Seed
Dose	$1/2$ teaspoon per cup
	Tincture 2ml, 1-2 times daily
Constituents	Volatile oil, alkaloids, bitters
Primary actions	Hormonal balancer
Secondary actions	Anti-spasmodic
	Diuretic
How it works	The 'chaste' aspects of the herb refer to its effects on men, where it has a noted sexual sedative quality. Its other name was monk's pepper! Its volatile oil acts on the pituitary gland and its connections with the hypothalamus, increasing dopamine effects in that area. It also increases the activity of luteinising hormone, so increases both progesterone and oestrogen production in the ovary, and it is noted for reducing excessive prolactin. This is what accounts for the hormone balancing effect, and its

traditional use for PMT symptoms, such as breast tenderness and bloating. The diuretic effect is probably also due to the volatile oil, and contributes to the relief of water retention and bloating. The bitters stimulate digestion, improving fat metabolism and nutrient absorption.

Growing guide   Fairly easy from seed under glass, needs a protected site in full sun.

False unicorn root

Latin name   Chamaelirium luteum
Origin   North America
Part used   Rhizome
Dose $1/2$ teaspoon per cup
Tincture 2ml, 1-3 times daily
Constituents   Bitters, steroidal saponins (including diosgenin), resin
Primary actions   Uterine tonic
Hormonal agent
Secondary actions   Anti-spasmodic
How it works   The saponins are similar in structure to female hormones, especially diosgenin which is a direct precursor of oestrogen. False unicorn root has a reputation for helping colic and flatulence. This action may be due to its bitters, which improve digestion, enhancing metabolism and absorption of nutrients. Its main use is in preventing miscarriage and vomiting in pregnancy as it

improves the function of the ovary. The same actions relieve general debility in menopause.

Caution   The fresh root may not be used as it can cause stupefaction and dizziness, these effects are lost on drying. This plant is in danger of being over-collected, so should only be used when all else has failed. There are plenty of similar hormone remedies to choose from. Herbalists are trying to establish cultivated sources.

Hops

Latin name	Humulus lupulus
Origin	Europe
Part used	Strobiles (flowers)
Dose	1 teaspoon to 1 cup
	Tincture 2ml, 3 times daily
Constituents	Volatile oil, bitter resin, tannins, valerianic acid, oestrogenic compounds, flavonoids
Primary actions	Sedative
	Hormonal agent
Secondary actions	Bitter digestive tonic
	Diuretic
How it works	Hops are very bitter, this helps to preserve beer, by inhibiting bacteria.the same action reduces fermentation and wind in the gut. The bitter-tasting compounds stimulate the production of bile in the liver. This action helps to prevent and relieve gallstones. The flavonoids are diuretic (promote the

elimination of water), so they relieve water retention, and the same group of chemicals contains oestrogenic substances which help to regulate periods. It is a useful relaxant nervine for irritability and for women who are at risk of developing gallstones. It is also possible that moderate, quality beer-drinking may be of benefit to menopausal women!

Growing guide   Very easy from layered cuttings, prefers sun and is a rampant climber.

Motherwort

Latin name	Leonurus cardiaca
Origin	Europe
Part used	Leaf and flower
Dose	1 teaspoon to 1cup
	Tincture 4ml, 3 times daily
Constituents	Alkaloids, bitter glycosides, flavonoids, caffeic acid, volatile oil
Primary actions	Sedative nervine
	Relaxing circulatory tonic
Secondary actions	Anti-spasmodic
	Uterine tonic
How it works	Motherwort offers an example of synergistic actions. The alkaloids, glycosides and flavonoids work together to reduce smooth (internal) muscle spasm, including the muscles of the heart, as its Latin name suggests. The alkaloids have a relaxing effect on the brain, so a feeling of calm results.

Together these actions relieve heart palpitations and nervous tension in menopause. Motherwort's name gives away its traditional use as a uterine tonic. 'Mother' is the old name for womb. It prepares the womb for easier contractions during labour and helps to reduce fibroid proliferation. It is not known which chemicals are responsible for these actions, but the general effect makes us assign it to the progesteronic group when mixing herbs for balance.

Growing guide   Tolerates most soils, prefers chalk, seeds itself in gardens.

Red Clover

Latin name	Trofolium pratense
Origin	Europe
Part used	Flowers
Dose	1 teaspoon per cup
	Tincture 4ml, 3 times daily
Constituents	Flavonoids, isoflavones, phenolic and cyanogenic glycosides, coumarins
Primary actions	Depurative
	Hormonal agent
Secondary actions	Anti-spasmodic
	Diuretic
	Anti-thrombotic circulatory tonic
How it works	The flavonoids are diuretic, so help the kidneys eliminate water and soluble toxins. This may account for red clover's traditional

use as a depurative in skin conditions. The phenols are antibiotic, so add to the cleansing effect on the skin. Coumarins reduce the stickiness of blood cells called platelets, which helps to prevent clots forming and causing thrombosis. Isoflavones are now known to be responsible for the hormonal action as they mimic oestrogen and provide precursors for oestrogen production. This explains the use of red clover tea to relieve hot flushes. Its oestrogenic effects contribute to heart and bone health in the menopause. Cyanogenic glycosides and coumarins are also anti-spasmodic as they relax smooth muscle, which can lower blood pressure a little by allowing blood vessels to dilate.

Caution	Not to be taken with other anti-clotting medication, such as Warfarin and Heparin.
Growing guide	Easy from seed, rather invasive, prefers sun.

Sage

Latin name	Salvia officinalis
Origin	Europe
Part used	Leaf
Dose	1 teaspoon per cup, Tincture 4ml, 3x daily
Constituents	Volatile oil, flavonoids, phenols, tannins, oestrogenic, saponins
Primary actions	Antiseptic

	Antibiotic
	Astringent
	Hormonal agent
Secondary actions	Digestive stimulant
	Anti-spasmodic
	Relaxant

How it works   The tannins and phenols act together to subdue bacteria on direct contact in the mouth and throat and is used as a wash for infected skin. The phenols also act in the gut to reduce bacterial fermentation, so they relieve wind. It is likely that the antibiotic phenols are responsible for sage's reputation for relieving night sweats in tuberculosis. and glandular fever. The bitters stimulate digestion of nutrients, especially fats, hence its use with rich meat and nut dishes. The hormonal compounds relieve hot flushes as well as night sweats, and reduce milk secretion so help when weaning infants. New research into the essential oils has confirmed its mildly relaxing qualities and shown its ability to improve mental function in the elderly. This is a supreme herb for women in menopause, as it relieves hot flushes and indigestion, relaxes and improves the mind!

Growing guide   Very tolerant of soils, prefers a sunny spot, easy from seed under glass.

Shepherd's purse

Latin name	Capsella bursa-pastoris
Origin	Europe
Part used	Leaf
Dose	1 teaspoon per cup
	Tincture 4ml, 3 times daily
Constituents	Flavonoids, polypeptides(including histamine, choline, acetylcholine), fumaric, bursic acid
Primary actions	Anti-haemorrhagic
	Astringent
Secondary actions	Urinary antiseptic
	Diuretic
How it works	The main action is probably due to the polypeptides' effect on the gut and the womb lining. They reduce proliferation and secretion of cells. This astringent action appears to reduce the growth of fibroids and prevents heavy bleeding from the womb, and inhibits diarrhoea in the gut. The flavonoids stabilise capillary walls, which contributes to the anti-haemorrhagic effect and circulatory health. The same chemical compounds may account for its traditional use in urinary infections, where blood loss from inflamed tissues in cystitis and kidney stones is prevented. Modern herbalists mainly prescribe shepherd's purse for heavy periods and bleeding from fibroids.
Growing guide	Sown from seed directly, seeds itself annually.

Squaw vine

Latin name	Mitchella repens
Origin	North America
Part used	Root and leaf
Dose	1 teaspoon per cup
	Tincture 4ml, 3 times daily
Constituents	Mucilage, tannins, saponins, resin
Primary actions	Uterine tonic
Secondary actions	Diuretic
How it works	Although its main use is to help the muscles of the womb in labour and birth, squaw vine is noted for its effect on heavy menstrual bleeding and painful periods. It is likely that the saponins are close to female hormones in structure, and responsible for its main effect. It also has a reputation for helping with exhaustion and irritability in both sexes and for relieving urinary infections. It isn't known which constituents have these effects.

White deadnettle

Latin name	Lamium album
Origin	Europe
Part used	Leaf
Dose	1 teaspoon per cup
	Tincture 4ml, 3 times daily
Constituents	Tannins, polypeptides (amines), flavonoids, alkaloids, saponins, mucilage
Primary actions	Astringent
	Uterine tonic

Secondary actions	Anti-spasmodic
	Prostate remedy
How it works	The polypeptides are probably responsible for this herb's ability to check heavy bleeding in menstruation and when applied to wounds topically. The saponins are likely to be hormonal and account for the anti-spasmodic and co-ordinating effects on uterine (womb) muscle. This is another herb to use in combination for women with heavy menstrual bleeding or fibroids.
Growing guide	From seed sown directly in spring

Wild yam

Latin name	Dioscorea villosa
Origin	South America
Part used	Rhizome
Dose	1 teaspoon per cup
	Tincture 4ml, 3 times daily
Constituents	Steroidal saponins, alkaloids, tannins, phytosterols
Primary actions	Anti-spasmodic
	Hormonal agent
Secondary actions	Digestive tonic
	Anti-inflammatory
How it works	It isn't known which constituents provide the anti-spasmodic action, which for many years was considered to be its main action, relieving colic and constipation. When modern research revealed the hormonal

action of the saponins and other phytosterols, wild yam became a favoured remedy for oestrogen deficiency in menopause. It also has a strong reputation for relieving arthritic stiffness and pain. This action may be due to the phytosterols (plant hormones). This plant was used to synthesise oestradiol when the contraceptive pill was first manufactured.

Growing guide   Not tried in Britain, poly tunnels might enable it to grow.

CIRCULATORY TONICS

Note If you are suffering from hot flushes and night sweats, you will find the spicy circulatory tonics, (ginger, chilli, mustard, horseradish) can make your symptoms worse, so to deal with circulatory problems you will need herbs which are not diaphoretic (sweat-inducing).

Gingko	Motherwort
Hawthorn	Passionflower (see Relaxants)
Horsechestnut	Rue

Ginkgo

Latin name	Ginkgo biloba
Origin	Asia
Part used	Leaf
Dose	1 teaspoon per cup
	Tincture 4ml, 3 times daily
Constituents	Ginkgolides, flavonoids

Primary actions	Circulatory tonic
Secondary actions	Anti-inflammatory
How it works	Research on ginkgo is growing, but little is known of its main chemical constituents. The ginkgolides stop blood cells called platelets from sticking together, so this provides the anti-thrombotic effect. Platelet aggregation also occurs in allergic reactions, so ginkgo is used in asthma and hayfever. Flavonoids are also noted for their stabilising effect on blood vessel walls, so this might be another reason why ginkgo inhibits inflammation (where water escapes from the leaky blood vessels and causes swelling). Its main reputation, newly arrived in Europe from the far East, is for improving circulation to the brain. Modern research has confirmed this effect. The flavonoids and ginkgolides probably act together to dilate and repair blood vessels, so help to protect against strokes. One study showed that it only had these effects in elderly people and showed no effect in younger men and women!
Caution	Not to be used with anti-coagulant medication such as Warfarin or Heparin.
Growing guide	Parks and estates only, as it is a very tall tree. Very tolerant of modern pollution.

Hawthorn

Latin name	Crataegus oxyacanthoides
Origin	Europe
Part used	Fruits
Dose	1 teaspoon per cup
	Tincture 2ml, 3 times daily
Constituents	Alkaloids, flavonoids, cyanogenic glycosides, saponins, tannins, phenols
Primary actions	Heart tonic
Secondary actions	Anti-spasmodic
	Diuretic
How it works	The flavonoids and glycosides improve the heart muscle's ability to use oxygen and reduce the fragility of small blood vessels. They are anti-spasmodic and mildly relaxing, so they dilate the blood vessels a little, which lowers blood pressure, and they help to stabilise the heart rate. The saponins are mildly anti-coagulant so reduce the tendency to thrombosis. When taken fresh the berries contain vitamin C, which aids the repair of blood vessel walls and keeps them smooth, so hindering plaque and damage from cholesterol deposits. Used as a gargle, the phenols and tannins are useful for sore throats. One of the alkaloids, amygdalin, is now called laetrile and has a new reputation as an anti-cancer agent. The flowers have some of the actions of the berries and can also be made into a tea.

Caution	Not to be taken with anti-clotting medication (such as Warfarin, Heparin, etc)or anti-arythmic drugs (Digoxin).
Growing guide	Will tolerate impossible conditions! Wild, wet and windy landscapes as well as urban streets. A very undervalued tree.

Horsechestnut

Latin name	Aesculus hippocastanum
Origin	Europe, Asia
Part used	Fruit, bark
Dose	1 teaspoon per cup
	Tincture 4ml, 1-3 times daily
Constituents	Saponins, tannins, glycosides, coumarins, tiglic, angelic acid, flavones
Primary actions	Venous tonic
	Astringent
Secondary actions	Diuretic
	Anti-inflammatory
How it works	The flavonoids and glycosides are deposited in the blood vessel walls, so improve their strength and elasticity. They are diuretic, so the extra elimination of water contributes to the reduction in swelling (oedema) which often accompanies weak, bulging (varicose) veins.The coumarins and saponins reduce clotting, so protect against thrombosis. The glycosides and flavones also inhibit the inflammatory process, so help to relieve phlebitis. Applied topically, tannins also

reduce bacterial infection as well as inflammation so are useful to treat leg ulcers. The acids are probably febrifuge (reduce temperature) as well as being mildly relaxant. This may account for the traditional use of horsechestnut in fevers.

Caution	Not to be taken with anti-coagulant medication, such as Warfarin, Heparin etc.
Growing guide	Only suitable for estate and park gardening, easy to germinate.

Motherwort

(see Hormonal agents).

Passionflower

(see Relaxants).

Rue

Latin name	Ruta graveolens
Origin	Europe
Part used	Leaf
Dose	1/2 teaspoon per cup
	Tincture 2ml, 1-3 times daily
Constituents	Volatile oil, flavonoids, coumarins, alkaloids, acids, phenols
Primary action	Anti-inflammatory
Secondary action	Anti-spasmodic
How it works	The volatile oil contains anti-spasmodic and anti-septic compounds, which help to relax and repair blood vessel walls. The flavonoids

also relax blood vessels and reduce their leakiness which inhibits inflammation. Coumarins are anti-coagulant, so help to protect against thrombosis. The main action of the alkaloids isn't known, they may be responsible for its reputation in relieving palpitations. When the herb is applied topically it reduces pain, this action is probably due to the volatile oil.

Caution   Some people are highly allergic to this plant, and develop severe blistering on contact. They are very few, but you should try a small skin patch test with your remedy first. Not to be taken with anti-coagulant medication Warfarin, Heparin etc.

Growing guide   From seed under glass, needs full sun.

IRON TONICS

Couch grass	Parsley	Yellow dock
Nettles	Watercress	

Couch Grass

Latin name	Triticum repens
Origin	Europe
Part used	Rhizome
Dose	1 teaspoon per cup
	Tincture 5ml, 1-3 times daily
Constituents	Mannitol, gum, muculage, volatile oil,

	vanillin, saponin, iron, minerals, vitamin B
Primary actions	Diuretic
	Demulcent
Secondary actions	Anti-biotic
	Iron tonic
How it works	Mannitol is a simple starch which tastes sweet but can't be used or stored for energy, so it has no calorific value. This type of sugar is an osmotic diuretic, (it eliminates water by pulling it along into the urinary tubules). Its mucilage is mildly antibiotic and demulcent and this also survives into the urinary system, soothing and healing inflamed surfaces in cystitis. Couch grass also has a traditional reputation for relieving liver and gallbladder problems, including gallstones and jaundice. It isn't known which constituents are responsible, but the saponins may play a role as they are known to break down fats and alter the permeability of cell walls. This grass has a high iron content so can be used when water retention and iron deficiency occur together.
Growing guide	Plant cut pieces just under soil. Highly invasive. Most people struggle to get rid of it!

Nettles

Latin name	Urtica dioica
Origin	Europe and world-wide
Part used	Leaf

Dose	1 teaspoon per cup
	Tincture 4ml, 1-3 times daily
Constituents	Indoles (including histamine, serotonin), potassium, iron, silica, trace minerals, tannins, acetylcholine,flavones, formic acid
Primary actions	Iron tonic
	Anti-inflammatory
	Anti-haemorrhagic
Secondary actions	Depurative
	Diuretic
	Hypo-glycaemic
How it works	The indoles and flavones are anti-inflammatory. This action applies to all types of inflammation, including asthma and eczema. It can relieve the pain of gout, arthritis and rheumatism. The diuretic effect of the flavones supports this action by removing waste metabolites from the joints and blood. The tannins and silica are probably responsible for its ability to stop bleeding, the tea can be applied to bleeding surfaces. Traditionally the tea was drunk to improve milk production in nursing mothers, although it is not known to have hormonal action. The fresh leaf may be cooked as a vegetable. (See Chapter 7).
Growing guide	Wearing rubber gloves, bury small sections of root just under the soil. Prefers damps soil, tolerates semi-shade.

Parsley

Latin name	Petroselinum crispum
Origin	Europe
Part used	Leaf
Dose	1 teaspoon per cup
	Tincture 4ml, 1-3 times daily
Constituents	Volatile oil, flavonoids, coumarins, minerals including iron, fresh leaf has Vitamins A and C
Primary actions	Carminative
	Diuretic
Secondary actions	Iron tonic
	Uterine stimulant
How it works	The volatile oil contains a number of constituents which reduce bacterial fermentation and muscular spasm in the gut. This is what is called a carminative action, which relieves wind and bloating. The coumarins are also anti-spasmodic and mildly anti-coagulant, so relax blood vessels and protect against thrombosis. The flavonoids are diuretic (increase elimination of water). Parsley is rich in iron and the fresh plant contains vitamin C which enhances iron absorption (see Chapter 7). It is a very good herb for menopausal women who suffer from water retention and iron deficiency anaemia, but not to be used in large quantities in pregnancy.
Growing guide	Difficult to germinate, likes hot, sandy soil,

doesn't transplant well. Sow seed in small,
sand filled trench under cloche in open
ground.

Watercress

(see Chapter 6).

Yellow dock

Latin name	Rumex crispus
Origin	Europe
Part used	Root
Dose	1 teaspoon per cup
	Tincture 4ml, 1-3 times daily
Constituents	Tannins, anthraquinone glycosides, bitters, iron, oxalates
Primary actions	Depurative
	Laxative
Secondary actions	Iron tonic
	Liver tonic
How it works	Anthraquinone glycosides cause the bowel wall to move, increasing the rate of elimination. Their effect is tempered by tannins, so it is not a strong laxative and doesn't cause griping. Bitters stimulate the liver's production of bile and its release from the gallbladder. This action also helps to emulsify fats and keeps the contents of the bowel soft. It is mainly used as a cleanser in skin complaints, athritis and rheumatism. You would generally choose this herb when

iron deficiency anaemia was also a problem. It has some reputation for inhibiting the growth of cancers in the digestive system.

Caution	Can make gout more painful, not to be used in pregnancy.
Growing guide	Self seeds and is difficult to eradicate. Tolerates any soil.

RELAXANTS

Black cohosh	Kava-kava	Skullcap
Chamomile	Lemon balm	Valerian
Cowslips	Limeflowers	Vervein
Cramp bark	Passionflower	Wild yam

Black Cohosh

(see Hormonal agents).

Chamomile

Latin name	Matricaria recutita (this plant has been renamed several times recently, so you must specify small, cone-headed flowers with single row of petals. This is currently called German chamomile)
Origin	Europe
Part used	Flowers
Dose	1 teaspoon per cup, 1-3 cups per day Tincture 5ml, 1-3 times daily
Constituents	Volatile oil, flavonoids, coumarins, valerianic

	acid, sesquiterpene bitters, salicylates, tannins
Primary action	Relaxant
Secondary actions	Anti-spasmodic
	Digestive tonic
How it works	Chamomile is one of the most complex herbs in common use. It has a little of almost every action shown by plants.The volatile oil acts on the brain to reduce sensitivity as well as being mildly antiseptic and anti-inflammatory when applied topically. Flavonoids are mildly diuretic, coumarins relax visceral muscle by acting on local nerve centres. The volatile oil is carminative (reduces bacterial ferment and wind in the gut).Sesquiterpene bitters stimulate bile production in the liver and there are bitter glycosides which add to this action. Anti-inflammatory salicylates are present in small quantities. Tannins astringe and tone the wall of the gut, alleviating diarrhoea.
Growing guide	Annual. Sow seeds each year in pots, window boxes or scatter freely in a sunny position in spring.

Cowslips

Latin name	Primula veris
Origin	Europe
Part used	Flowers
Dose	$1/2$ teaspoon per cup
	Tincture 2ml, 1-3 times daily

Constituents	Saponins, volatile oil, flavonoids, phenols, tannins, glycosides
Primary actions	Sedative
	Anti-spasmodic
Secondary actions	Expectorant
How it works	The saponins are expectorant as they increase the production of thin mucus which relieves bronchial tubes from congestion by thick, sticky mucus. The phenols are mildy antibiotic. The anti-spasmodic effect is mainly due to the flavonoids and the glycosides which are similar to aspirin compounds. The cowslip has a very long, traditional use for nervous irritability and headaches as well as paralytic ailments (perhaps these were of the nervous variety?). It can be used for all cases of restlessness, especially if you have a tendency to bronchitis or asthma.
Caution	Being over-collected in the wild, buy only cultivated stock.
Growing guide	Easy-to-grow from seed under glass, plant out in spring, prefers damp soil.

Cramp Bark

Latin name	Viburnum opulus
Origin	Europe
Part used	Bark
Dose	1 teaspoon per cup 1-3 cups per day
	Tincture 3ml, 1-3 times daily

Constituents	Viburnine, tannin, valerianic acid, coumarins
Primary action	Anti-spasmodic
Secondary actions	Relaxant
	Digestive tonic
How it works	Coumarins and other constituents relax muscle by reducing the number of messages sent to the brain. They affect both digestive muscle and skeletal muscle. Valerianic acid acts on the brain to reduce reception of messages, producing a feeling of relaxation. Viburnine is bitter, so has a tonic effect on digestion. The tannins reduce the free flow of water through the gut wall, so help to alleviate diarrhoea.
Caution	Some people feel drowsy when they take this herb, so wait one hour after drinking for the first time to see what effect it has on you before driving or operating machinery.
Growing guide	Easy-to-grow shrub, green-white flower heads in early spring, available in most garden centres as snowball bush.

Kava-kava

Latin name	Piper methysticum
Origin	South Sea Islands
Part used	Root
Dose	1 teaspoon per cup, 1-2 cups per day
	Tincture 3ml, 1-2 times daily
Constituents	Pyrones, piperidine alkaloids, glycosides, mucilage

Main actions	Relaxant
	Anti-depressant
Secondary actions	Anti-spasmodic
	Diuretic
How it works	Not much is known about the actions of Kava-kava, though research is increasing as it becomes popular. The pyrones and piperidines act centrally (on the brain) to reduce sensitivity to pain. Applied topically it is rubefacient and numbing. It also has a reputation for relieving fatigue, so in some books it is referred to as a stimulant. It is best to view it like alcohol, relaxing and stimulating at the same time, with some effects of intoxication at high doses.
Growing guide	Not possible in the British Isles.

Lemon balm

Latin name	Melissa officinalis
Origin	Europe
Part used	Leaf
Dose	1 teaspoon per cup 1-3 cups per day
	Tincture 4ml, 1-3 times daily
Constituents	Volatile oil, flavonoids, phenols, triterpenes, tannins
Primary actions	Relaxant
	Digestive tonic
Secondary actions	Anti-viral
	Anti-thyroid
How it works	The volatile oil has a central relaxing effect

(on the brain) as well as reducing thyroid hormone stimulation of other systems. It also inhibits the growth of viruses such as herpes by giving a sort of repellant protection to the tissues, and possibly penetrating viral coating. The phenols add to this effect and help to dispel bacteria in the gut. Triterpenes are bitter, so stimulate digestive secretions. Tannins astringe the wall of the gut, alleviating diarrhoea.

Growing guide   You will rarely have to resort to seed, nearly everyone has some lemon balm to give away, it seeds itself like mad, tolerates any soil and will grow in pots.

Limeflowers

Latin name	Tilia europaea
Origin	Europe
Part used	Leaf and flower
Dose	1 teaspoon per cup, 1-2 cups per day
	Tincture 4ml, 1-3 times daily
Constituents	Volatile oil, flavonoids, phenols, mucilage, tannins
Primary actions	Relaxant
	Lowers blood pressure
Secondary actions	Increases sweating
	Anti-spasmodic
How it works	The volatile oil reduces the brain's sensitivity to pain messages. Mucilage soothes stomach and gut wall and flavonoids make blood

vessels less fragile. Phenols are antiseptic and diaphoretic (increase sweating), which induces dilation of blood vessels. The overall effect is to calm and lower blood pressure. Limeflowers is a particularly nice tasting tea.

Growing guide   Too large for the average garden, a most magnificent specimen can be seen at Kew Gardens in London.

Passionflower

Latin name	Passiflora incarnata
Origin	America
Part used	Leaf
Dose	1 teaspoon per cup, 1-2 cups per day
	Tincture 2 ml, 1-2 times daily
Constituents	Alkaloids, saponins, flavonoids
Primary actions	Relaxant (mental and muscular)
	Anti-spasmodic
Secondary action	Pain reliever

How it works   Alkaloids act on the brain, reducing sensitivity to pain. The alkaloids in passionflower are known to work on nerves in the spinal cord which control the movement of blood vessels and digestive muscles. This produces a relaxing effect which lowers blood pressure. The flavonoids supplement vitamin C in strengthening blood vessels.

Growing guide   An easy-to-grow climber but needs a south-facing wall or fence.

Skullcap

Latin name	Scutellaria laterifolia
Origin	America
Part used	Leaf
Dose	1 teaspoon per cup, 1-2 cups per day
	Tincture 3ml, 1-3 times daily
Constituents	Flavonoids, glycosides, iridoids, volatile oil, tannin
Primary action	Relaxant
Secondary actions	Anti-spasmodic
	Possibly anti- inflammatory
How it works	Little is known about the active constituents of American skullcap as most research is based on a Chinese variant. We rely on the tradition of use for our knowledge of its actions. The anti-inflammatory effect is present in the Chinese variety and it is very likely that both varieties have the same constituents. American skullcap is noted for its central (brain) calming effect, flavonoids stabilise blood vessel walls and contribute to its mooted anti-inflammatory effect, as well as mildly increasing the elimination of water via the kidneys. It has a long traditional use for neurological diseases such as epilepsy and motor neurone diseases.
Growing guide	Prefers damp soil, sow under glass and plant out in early summer in a warm, damp spot (pond-side, bog-garden).

Valerian

Latin name	Valeriana officinalis
Origin	Europe
Part used	Root
Dose	1 teaspoon per cup, one cup per night
	Tincture 2-5ml, nightly
Constituents	Valerianic acid, alkaloids, glycosides, tannins, choline, flavonoids, valepotriates, iridoids
Primary action	Relaxant/sedative
Secondary action	Anti-spasmodic
How it works	Valerianic acid and valepotriates reduce excitability of brain and feelings of anxiety. Best used at night as it is on the borderline between relaxants and sedatives. Flavonoids are mildly diuretic (increase water elimination).
Growing guide	Sow directly in a sunny spot with damp soil in early spring.

Vervein

Latin name	Verbena officinalis
Origin	Europe
Part used	Leaf, flower
Dose	1 teaspoon per cup, 1-3 cups per day
	Tincture 3ml,1-3 times daily
Constituents	Glycosides, iridoids, bitters, volatile oil, alkaloids, mucilage
Primary actions	Relaxant
	Bitter digestive tonic
Secondary actions	Anti-depressant

	Anti-viral
	Febrifuge
How it works	Not all actions are clearly understood. Bitters stimulate liver and digestive secretions, unknown constituents act on the brain to reduce sensitivity to pain and increase feelings of well-being. These are probably found in the volatile oil, which is responsible for the anti-viral effect, acting as a repellant in the tissues of the body. This is known as the 'constitutional effect' which French aromatherapists call the 'terrain theory'. The whole herb has some pain relieving action when applied as a poultice to inflamed joints and muscles.

Wild yam

(see Hormonal agents).

DIGESTIVE TONICS

Agrimony	Rosemary	Wormwood
Chamomile	Sage	
Gentian	Thyme	

Agrimony

Latin name	Agrimonia eupatoria
Origin	Europe
Part used	Leaf

Dose	1 teaspoon per cup
	Tincture 2ml, 1-3 times daily
Constituents	Volatilie oil, tannins, coumarins, flavonoids, polysaccharides, silica
Primary actions	Digestive tonic
	Astringent
Secondary actions	Anti-viral
	Wound-healer
How it works	The tannins and volatile oil are probably responsible for Agrimony's use as a gargle and antiseptic wound dressing. They continue their antibacterial action in the gut, where they reduce fermentation, relieving wind and bloating. The polysaccharides, together with volatile oil, may also be anti-viral by preventing access to cells and increasing immune response. The bitter compounds stimulate production of bile, which aids digestion of fats and improves bowel function. The coumarins relax gallbladder muscle to allow free flow of bile into the gut. The tannins help to reduce leakiness of gut walls, so may reduce sensitivity to troublesome foods. Flavonoids improve the strength of the small blood vessels, so help the gut lining to be less inflamed. Agrimony is a good herb for women with sensitive digestion and a tendency to gallstones or acid reflux.
Growing guide	2ft high perennial, very tolerant of poor, dry soil.

Chamomile

(See Relaxants).

Gentian

Latin name	Gentiana lutea
Origin	Europe
Part used	Root
Dose	1/2 teaspoon per cup
	Tincture 2ml, 1-3 times daily
Constituents	Bitter glycosides, flavonoids, phenols, alkaloids, mono-saccharides
Primary actions	Liver tonic
	Digestive tonic
Secondary actions	Antiseptic
	Uterine stimulant
How it works	The bitter taste gives the main effect to this herb – it causes a reflex production of digestive secretions and bile from the liver, which aids breakdown and absorption of nutrients. Bile acids keep the content of the bowel soft and increase regular movement of the bowel muscle known as peristalsis. The phenols are antiseptic and mildly antibiotic, so help to reduce bacterial fermentation in the gut, relieving wind and bloating.
Growing guide	Needs a sunny, well drained rockery or Alpine meadows!

Rosemary

Latin name	Rosemarinus officinalis
Origin	Europe
Part used	Leaf (oil externally)
Dose	1 teaspoon per cup, 1-2 cups per day
	Tincture 3ml, 1-3 times daily
Constituents	Volatile oil, phenols, flavonoids, tannins,
	bitters, resin
Primary actions	Digestive tonic
	Circulatory tonic
Secondary actions	Anti-inflammatory
	Carminative
How it works	The volatile oil contains several compounds

The volatile oil contains several compounds which stimulate nerve endings and produce a sense of warmth. They also stimulate the lining of the digestive system, which responds by secreting more digestive juices. The bitters stimulate the liver to produce more bile, so that fatty meat and nut dishes are more easily digested (hence the famous combination of Rosemary and lamb). The phenols are mildly antiseptic, they reduce fermentation in the gut, alleviating wind and colic. The volatile oil components penetrate brain tissue, where they facilitate nerve message transmission. This action has given rise to the traditional view that Rosemary improves memory. Research trials using oils of Sage and Rosemary with elderly residents of nursing homes have shown it to reliably

| | improve mental function. |
| *Growing guide* | Easy from cuttings in sandy compost, doesn't like cold winds. |

Sage

(See Hormonal agents).

Thyme

Latin name	Thymus vulgaris
Origin	Europe
Part used	Leaf
Dose	1 teaspoon per cup
	Tincture 4ml, 1-3 times daily
Constituents	Volatile oil, bitters, saponins, phenols, flavonoids, tannins
Primary actions	Antibiotic
	Bitter
Secondary actions	Carminative
	Astringent
How it works	Bitters produce effects described above (see gentian), increasing bowel movement and absorption of nutrients. Thyme oil is strongly antiseptic and the tannins add to the antibacterial effect when applied directly to skin or digestive linings, so relieving wind and bloating. The flavonoids are anti-spasmodic so they reduce tension in the muscles of the gut. It is these two actions which provide the carminative effect. Saponins help to emulsify fats and facilitate

secretion and absorption of digestive fluids as well as helping the production of thin mucus in the bronchial tubes. Thyme is best known for its volatile oil, which reduces inflammation and infection in the respiratory system. Volatile oils are noted for diffusing through all tissues and can be breathed out via the lungs. Thyme's relief of bronchitis and asthma relies on this action.

Growing guide Easy to grow from seed under glass and cuttings in sandy soil. Prefers a sunny spot.

Wormwood

Latin name Artemisia absinthum
Origin Europe
Part used Leaf
Dose 1/3 teaspoon per cup
Tincture 2ml, 1-3 times daily
Constituents Volatile oil, bitters, phenols, tannins, coumarins
Primary actions Digestive tonic
Carminative
Secondary actions Uterine stimulant
Antiseptic
How it works Wormwood is the most bitter herb known in European medicine. It increases liver function, especially production of bile and digestive secretions. Phenols and tannins reduce bacterial fermentation and the volatile oil adds to this effect, which is strong enough

to remove intestinal worms. Flavonoids and the volatilie oil are anti-spasmodic, so the whole effect is to increase absorption and relieve wind or bloating. The Artemisia family has an additional hormonal effect which is not yet understood but has a beneficial effect on the uterus, being noted for helping female infertility. It is one of the best digestive tonics, especially useful for women with digestive infections such as candida.

Caution   Not to be used in pregnancy, where it may cause miscarriage.

5

Making your own herbal remedies

You can prepare herbs in a wide variety of ways to relieve menopausal problems.

Types of herbal preparation

Oral remedies:
- teas
- tinctures
- syrups
- pills

Topical applications:
- creams
- oils
- baths

Measurements
1ml= 1g ,1 teaspoon = 5ml, 1 cup = 165ml

Oral remedies

Doses for adults

Adult doses of tincture vary according to the herbs used in them. Usually 1/2 a teaspoon of single herb tinctures, three times daily, is required. With great care, you can get 80 drops onto a 5ml teaspoon, so you can work out your dose that way too, and use the formula given below to calculate a child's dose. The amount of alcohol is negligible, but you can add the remedy to hot water and allow some of the alcohol to evaporate if you wish.

Teas are usually drunk in doses of 1 teaspoon per cup, up to 3 cups per day.

Elderly people may require different doses, as body weight falls or if digestion isn't as good. One should start with a lower dose and work up if required.

These are much bigger doses than is often suggested on over-the-counter tincture bottles, where the manufacturer is more concerned with keeping the price and profit margin at an attractive level. Tinctures are more expensive than teas, and you should expect to pay between £3 and £5 for a week's supply.

Doses for children

Children require smaller doses. There are some formulae which can be used, based on a child's age. For example: divide the child's age by 20, to give the proportion of an adult dose, eg. 6 (years) divided by 20 = 3/10 adult dose. You also have to take into account the child's body weight, giving less if a child is underweight for his/her age. Common doses are; 1 tablespoon of tea to a child under 5, 1/2 a cup for a child from 5 to 10 years and a full cup from 11 years onwards.

Beatrice Potter seems to agree, as Peter Rabbit was given a large spoonful of Chamomile tea after he had over-eaten in Mr McGregor's garden.

Teas

Teas (also called tisanes) can be made directly from dried herbs. Leaves and flowers require five minutes steeping in freshly boiled water. Always place a saucer or cover on the cup to keep in valuable aromatic ingredients. This is known as an **infusion**. Roots, barks, seeds and berries need boiling for five minutes in a covered pan. This is called a **decoction**. The usual dose is 1 rounded teaspoon per cup (about 4g to 165ml). Regular use means 1 or 2 cups per day for several weeks. Infusions and decoctions can be drunk cold, and any flavouring can be added after steeping or boiling.

- To make an **infusion**, steep the cut leaves or flowers in boiling water for five to ten minutes.
- To make a **decoction**, boil cut root or bark on the stove for five to ten minutes.

Tinctures

Tinctures have become very popular in Britain, both among herbalists and consumers. They are made by soaking herbal material, finely chopped, in an alcoholic liquid, about 70% proof. This could be brandy or vodka. You generally use one part herb to five parts liquid, so 100g to 500ml. Chop the herbs as finely as possible and cover with the alcohol. Turn, shake or stir every day for ten days. This is to ensure that every particle of herb is in contact with alcohol, otherwise moulds may develop. After 10 days, strain and squeeze out the remaining 'marc' through a clean piece of material. Keep the tincture you have made in a dry bottle with a tight stopper.

This can be used in place of herbal tea. Each teaspoon of tincture generally gives the effect of a small cup of tea. Sometimes herbal constituents are extracted better by alcohol, so it is a useful way of preserving herbs. In the past wines and vinegars were used, and their trace is found in the nursery rhyme Jack and Jill where 'Old Dame Dob did mend Jack's nob with vinegar and brown paper.'

Tincture of Lemon Balm
100g lemon balm
500ml vodka or brandy

Chop herbs finely, cover with alcohol, shake or stir daily for ten days, strain and bottle.

Syrups

Herbs can be preserved in syrup but they are quite difficult to make, as the proportion of sugar to herbal material is crucial. They frequently go mouldy however carefully you measure. There are two methods. The first is the simplest, but only keeps for a few days but this may be a useful recipe for children's ailments which often blow over quickly.

Syrup recipe 1

Place chopped herbs and sugar in 1cm layers in a clean, dry jar, finishing with a sugar layer. Leave for one day. You will find that a syrup has formed. You can shake the jar gently once a day until all the sugar has turned into syrup. This may take 3 days but you can use the product immediately.

Syrup recipe 2

Soak 4g of herb, finely chopped, in 56ml water for 12 hours. Strain and squeeze out the herbs. There should be about 45ml liquid. Add 90g sugar, stir over heat until dissolved, boil briefly, strain through a filter paper or cloth. You should have about 100ml syrup. This must be kept in a well stoppered bottle in a cool, dry, dark cupboard. The dose would usually be 1 teaspoon at a time for children, and a dessertspoon from 11 years onwards.

Pills, tablets and capsules

Pills and tablets are made by crushing herbs together with

binding agents. Capsules are filled with herbs. In both cases powdered herbs are used.

Capsules are usually made of gelatine, although vegetarian ones can be obtained. Most are of a standard size, containing about 2g of herb. You can buy herbs ready powdered and fill your own capsules by hand. It's a very sneezy, time consuming business! Tablets are made by pressing powdered herbs into the required shape. You will need to add ingredients to make the dough stick together and the tablets hold their shape. Manufacturers usually use vegetable gums, but quite satisfactory tablets can be made at home using honey and arrowroot as binders. Pills can be pinched off and rolled between the fingers or tablets cut by hand from dough rolled with a pin.

Pill recipe
2 tablespoons buckwheat flour
1 tablespoon arrowroot
4 teaspoons runny honey

Knead all well together, add more honey if required. Dust board with arrowroot, roll out, cut to shape, dry overnight.

Topical remedies

Herbs can be applied to the outside of your body in several forms. This is known as topical application. You need first to know a little bit about skin in order to understand how herbs reach their target when used in this way.

Understanding how skin works

Skin has several layers designed to keep water in (you suffer dehydration quickly if large areas of skin are broken) but allow moisture out when required to cool the body down by evaporation. It is covered with a cornified layer (dead cells) and wax. Blood vessels are very close to the surface, and they **dilate** when we are hot, to allow heat out by convection. They also dilate when we are emotionally stressed, so we flush with anger, embarassment or affection. These blood vessels can **constrict** to conserve heat, and sometimes when we are very angry or upset, we become paler than our usual colour.

Fat underneath the skin keeps heat in by insulation and protects some areas from pressure (famously the bum!). Muscle is found underneath linings below the fatty layer. If you want to reach muscles, your topical applications must somehow get through the wax, cornified layer, fat and muscle linings first. Oily preparations do penetrate through these layers to some extent.

Increasing absorption through the skin

One way of increasing penetration is to soak the skin in water for a while. This can be done in the bath, in a steam room, or on small areas with a poultice or plaster.

Belladonna plasters for back pain could still be bought in the chemist's until a few years ago. Most people have heard of anti-smoking and hormone patches. These use the same principle. Back to Old Dame Dob and her vinegar on brown paper!

Essential oils can be added to the bath, a few drops in soap solution or a little milk to aid dispersal. This can be useful in aiding relaxation or soothing itchy, sore skin.

Oils

There are many essential oils available now which save you the time involved in infusing plants in oil, but this option is still valid if you want to use herbs from your garden.

Making an infused oil

Simply pick a handful of fresh herbs, chop finely and cover loosely with any oil – almond, olive or even sunflower. Place the bowl of oil and herbs in a pan of water and put the lid on. Heat until simmering and leave on the lowest possible heat for 1-2 hours. A slow-pot can give ideal conditions for making infused oils as it maintains a constant very low simmering temperature. Spices can also be used in infused oils.

Baths

Essential oils can be added to the bath for a relaxing effect – simply add five to ten drops of oil to your bath.

Infused oils can be added to the bath, which is an easy way of applying a very thin layer of soothing moisturiser to dry, itchy skin. One teaspoon of oil is usually enough. Beware, the bath will need extra cleaning afterwards, but no harm is done to bath surfaces.

Creams

These are more complicated to make. It would be easier to choose a favourite bland cream over the counter and add aromatic oils or tinctures as you wish. If you want to try a cream, try the following recipe.

Recipe for cream

8 parts oil
1 part beeswax
A few drops essential oil

Gently heat the oil and beeswax together in a bowl set in a pan of water on the stove. When the wax has melted, add the essential oil and pour into pots immediately.

Greasy ointments like this are generally not considered to be good for skin conditions such as eczema, where they inhibit healing and trap heat, but they are suitable for applying as muscle and joint rubs, as well as moisturising skin. Their advantage over liquid preparations is that they don't drip onto the carpets.

~ 6 ~

Choosing, growing and storing herbs

Identifying herbs

First it is important to know that you have the right plant. Some botanical families include poisonous and edible plants which look very similar and can only be distinguished from each other by fine botanical detail, like Hemlock and Valerian, which have subtle differences in stem and flower colouring. You could buy a field botany guide, as identification of plants is a great hobby, but it would be wiser not to select your remedies from the wild if you are a complete beginner.

Fortunately many of the most important medicinal herbs are garden favourites such as Thyme, Sage, Rosemary, Lemon balm and Peppermint. Most people recognise them and they are pretty unmistakeable. Even where there are different varieties, such as the Thymes and Mints, they have the same aroma and characteristics. It is better to choose the original sort for medicinal purposes rather than a variety because it may be a more reliable source of the chemicals that you need for your remedy.

Choosing herbs

There is a system of naming plants which gives each one two Latin names – the family name comes first and has a capital letter, the individual name comes second written in lower case. The meaning is reversed in Latin, for example *Thymus vulgaris* means common thyme. This is the one you would use for cough medicine. Other types, such as *Thymus aureus* (Golden Thyme) or *Thymus serpillus* (Creeping Thyme) will do no harm, but they don't have as much aroma – in fact they put most of their energy into looking pretty! The same can be said for the many lovely varieties of Achillea – a cottage garden flower related to yarrow (*Achillea officinalis*). The word *officinalis* in a plant's name means it was known to be used medicinally in the 17th century or before. You will need to specify both names when you are buying seeds or plants from nurseries. Addresses of reliable firms are given on page 140.

Growing herbs

Many of the herbs mentioned in this book can be grown in British gardens, some can be grown in pots or on window ledges. Growing herbs is a very relaxing and rewarding hobby. Although most aromatic herbs originate in the warm Mediterranean countries, they will do fine in a sunny spot in any garden soil, even on London clay.

They do prefer well drained, slightly dry soil, so adding grit and compost will help them along.

If you are growing from seed you will need to start them off in pots on a window ledge or in a greenhouse. To sow seeds really successfully you should buy John Innes compost number 1. This contains lots of sand and fine grit, so that water runs through quickly and the seed doesn't sit in its own tiny puddle of water, which causes a fungal growth gardeners call damping off.

When you have a small stem with two leaves, you pull it up gently and plant it in a pot with John Innes number 2 compost. This has more soil, so that fine roots can spread and take in water. It also contains a little more nutrient to feed the growing plant. When your plant is about 10 cm tall or has a few branches, it's time to plant it in a sunny spot or container, using John Innes number 3. John Innes is a type of compost, not a brand name, so you can ask for it in any nursery or garden department.

Planting out

Locate your herbs in the south-west corner of your garden if possible. Herbs don't need feeding or watering once they have extended their roots into the garden soil (after about a week) but containers will need to be watered as they dry out continually. You can even grow herbs in hanging baskets. You can use multipurpose compost, but you run a much greater risk of damping-off and losing seed before they even grow, which can mean a whole growing year lost. If your plants don't succeed in one spot in your garden, move them! Just dig up enough soil around the plant to ensure minimum root disturbance and put them in somewhere else. Experiment to see what works. There are plenty of herbs to choose from, so find one that suits your garden or space.

- Choose a sunny spot
- Add grit to improve drainage
- Start tender plants under glass
- Water pots and baskets daily
- Move plants if they aren't happy.

Harvesting and storing herbs

Choosing the right part of the plant

It is important to know which part of the plant you need if you are going to make your own herbal remedies. Flowers, leaves, roots, bark and berries are commonly used but sometimes one part of a plant is edible whereas another part is poisonous. We eat the tuberous root of the potato but avoid the berries, and we eat rhubarb stems but not the leaves. Comfrey root stores too many alkaloids, which can damage the liver, whereas they are barely present in the leaf. It is common to find stems in with leaves in herbs sold over the counter, as it is difficult to separate them when preparing herbs on a large scale. If you are preparing your own, you should take the trouble to rub the leaves off the stems as your remedy will be stronger without this inert woody matter.

Harvesting herbs

Choosing the right time to harvest is also important. It helps you to get the best quality of herbs in terms of the chemical constituents.

- Leaves are picked just before flowers develop
- Flowers are picked as they come out
- Berries as they become fully ripe, while they are still smooth and shiny
- Bark and stem is stripped in the late spring from new branches
- Roots are dug up in early autumn before the first frosts – pick on a dry day and scrub immediately after digging.

Storing herbs

Most plants can be used fresh, but it is more convenient to dry them for use all the year round.

The rules for drying herbs are; **as cool, fast, dark and dry as possible**, with as much air circulating around the individual herbs as can be allowed. The best way for home preservation is to hang up small bunches of herbs, loosely tied, in a dark room or shed. A washing-line strung across the attic is ideal. Hanging up in the kitchen will cause most of the colour and aroma to be lost before they dry.

Large roots should be chopped before drying, as they will prove too tough for the knife otherwise. They can be spread out in a single layer on newspapers. The newspapers should be changed when they feel very damp.

Herbal material is ready to store when it is **cracking dry**. This is a matter of experience, usually leaves will simply not leave their stems until they are thoroughly dry. Roots should snap briskly or fail to bend under pressure. Berries usually give a little under thumb pressure. They are slow to dry, and moulds develop if there is too much moisture, so gentle heat (airing cupboard level) is helpful.

When thoroughly dry, herbs should be stored in **cool, dark, dry, airless conditions** because sunlight destroys colour, air removes flavour and water causes moulds. Tin boxes are ideal, however plastic tubs and glass jars are OK provided they are kept in a cupboard.

- Hang leaves on branches upside down
- Spread roots out in a single layer
- Dry as fast as possible in a cool, dark, airy place
- Ready when cracking dry
- Keep in cool, dark, dry, airless conditions.

Fresh and dried herbs

Many people ask if the dosage of dried herbs should be different from fresh herbs. As the loss of chemicals in drying may balance the greater concentration due to loss of water, it is best to simply use the same amounts whether fresh or dry. Some herbs such as lemon balm, chamomile and basil taste better when fresh and are slightly more effective, but most herbs keep their medicinal properties very well if dried carefully. Roots and barks often improve their taste with drying, as they lose their acrid components and become sweeter.

❧ 7 ❧

Using nutrition for
a healthy menopause

How do we know what a healthy diet is? Governments in many countries produce guidelines, based on what it takes to prevent deficiencies and disease. Most of the British work on this was done in the years during and straight after World War Two. The way we eat has changed a great deal over the past 40 years, as new foods have arrived in Britain which were unheard of before the 1960s. American and Canadian government research gives us information on these 'new foods'. The result is a set of tables of what women, men and children with different lifestyles need to eat to stay free of deficiencies. Here we have presented figures for women doing sedentary or light physical work between the ages of 18-64.

- 1mg = one thousandth of 1g , 1µg = 1 millionth of 1g

Daily requirements for nutrients

Britsh research

Daily requirements for women 18-54	
kcals	2,150
protein	54g
calcium	500mg
iron	12mg
vitamin A	750µg
vitamin C	30mg
vitamin D	10µg if no sunlight available

American research

Daily requirements for women 18-54	
vitamin K	70-140µg
potassium	1,875-562mg
phosphorous	700-800mg
sodium	1,100-3,300
chloride	1,700-5,100

Canadian research

	25-49	over 50
vitamin E	6mg	
folacin (vitamin B)	175µg	190µg
pyridoxine (vitamin B_{12})	2µg	
magnesium	200mg	210mg
calcium	700mg	800mg
iodine	160µg	
zinc	8mg	

Special dietary needs of menopausal women

Asking women and their doctors what they should prioritise in menopause produces a shortlist:

- Energy
- Bones
- Hormones
- Heart health.

The suggested daily requirements for women change according to age and hormone status. As oestrogen levels diminish in the female body after menopause, bone density may lessen. Some researchers recommend increasing calcium intake at this time, but this doesn't increase the rate at which this mineral is deposited in the bones. American and Canadian dieticians recommend much higher calcium intakes than their British counterparts because the protein intake in these countries is generally higher, and this promotes the excretion of calcium from the body. Although it is sensible to eat sufficient calcium for one's daily needs, herbalists recommend:

- Optimising the digestive processes which increase the absorption of calcium
- Balancing hormones
- Exercising to ensure deposition in bones.

Calcium

Daily requirement 500g.

Used to give rigidity to bone.

You will find 500mg calcium in	Normal portion	Gives approximate % daily need
50g dried milk	10g	20%
70g cheddar cheese	50g	66%
100g tinned sardines	50g	50%
200g watercress	25g	12.5%
200g figs	25g	12.5%
250g carob flour	100g	50%

Maximising calcium absorption

- Combine with phosphorus (in peanuts, meat, cheese, onions, garlic, chocolate, carob)
- Have drinks and sauces containing orange, tomato etc. with meals
- Take vitamin D in fish oil, lentils
- Have digestive herbs in meals and drinks
- Avoid tea with meals
- Avoid high protein slimming diets.

B vitamins

These are necessary for every process in the body, including nerve transmission and protein building, as they are part of the process which turns sugar into fuel which every cell in the body needs to carry on its work. This affects nerve transmission, building structures such as muscle and bone, as well as making new 'fabrics' such as skin and mucus membranes. It is worth looking at these vitamins for energy and health, especially as some researchers think many people are deficient in them.

Thiamin

Vitamin B1, daily requirement 1.5mg.

Food	Amount per 100g	Normal portion	Approximate % of daily requirement
Brewers' yeast	15.6mg	10g	100%
Sunflower seeds	2mg	50g	66%
Pork	1mg	100g	66%
Green peas	.5mg	50g	16%
Wheatgerm	2g	10g	13%
Wholewheat bread	.34mg	25g	5%

Tea contains a small amount of thiamin, 1 cup is equivalent to a slice of wholemeal bread, but because of the quantities drunk in Britain it is a significant contributor to our thiamin intake.

Riboflavin

Vitamin B2, daily requirement 1.2mg.

Food	Amount per 100g	Normal portion	Approximate % of daily requirement
Liver	4.6mg	100g	400%
Almonds	.7mg	50g	29%
Marmite	11mg	3g	27%
Beefsteak	.23mg	100g	19%
Milk	.17mg	100ml	14%

Tea also contains a small amount of riboflavin, because of the amount we drink, this may be a significant contributor to our daily need.

Niacin

Vitamin B3, daily requirement 13g.

Food	Amount per 100g	Normal portion	Approximate % of daily requirement
Tuna	15.5mg	100g	119%
Peanuts	14.3mg	50g	111%
Liver	14.4mg	100g	111%
Chicken	5.9mg	100g	45%
Brewers' yeast	39mg	10g	29%
Mushrooms	4.4mg	50g	16%

Tea also contains good amounts of niacin, and can make an important contribition to our daily need. Niacin can be made in the body from tryptophan, which is present in cheese, fish, eggs and meat, with small amounts in bread, potatoes, brown rice and wheatgerm.

Folacin

Vitamin B₄, daily requirement 165 µg.

Food	Amount per 100g	Normal portion	Approximate % of daily requirement
Brewers' yeast	3912µg	10g	236%
Spinach	467µg	50g	141%
Sunflower seeds	236µg	50g	71%
Haricot beans	56.8µg	75g	25%
Broccoli	68.5µg	50g	20%
Wheatgerm	82µg	50g	24%

Dandelion leaf contains the same amount per 100g as wheatgerm.

Pyridoxine

Vitamin B₆, daily requirement .2mg.

Food	Amount per 100g	Normal portion	Approximate % of daily requirement
Salmon	.8mg	100g	40%
Sunflower seeds	1.2mg	50g	30%
Brewers' yeast	5mg	10g	25%
Banana	.51mg	75g	19%
Baked potato	.25mg	150g	18%
Beefsteak	.27mg	100g	13%

Carob flour is reported to have very large amounts of B6 but the data is not confirmed.

Biotin and Pantothenic acid

These are also B vitamins, but they are not normally included in detailed tables because they occur in almost all foods and deficiencies are unknown.

Cobalamine

Vitamin B_{12}, daily requirement 2-3µg.
The trace of vitamin B_{12} in food is so small that no detailed figures are available. It was once thought that you could only obtain this essential vitamin from animal foods, but recent research shows it to be present in pulses, such as mung beans, peas, alfalfa and soya beans. Comfrey leaf and whole wheat are also thought to provide useful amounts, though Comfrey is usually taken in short courses of eight weeks, with breaks between, as its alkaloids can accumulate in the liver. Consult a medical herbalist for more information on this.

How do you ensure the right amount of B vitamins in your diet?

You should eat **enough from each group** to supply your daily requirement. B vitamins are water soluble so you should use the minimum water to cook your foods, and keep the water to make sauce or gravy. The figures presented here give fairly large portions for meat and small for nuts or vegetables. This is based on general eating habits as represented in statistics. You can do the reverse, vegetarians and vegans would do this anyway. You must always aim to take a balance of B vitamins, as excesses or deficiencies in one can disturb the effect of the others.

How to increase B vitamins in your diet

Increases in this list refer to normal portions in the tables above.

- Add brewers' yeast to drinks, soups and sauces
- Eat more liver flavoured with tomato or orange
- Add wheatgerm to your breakfast cereal
- Add sunflower seeds to breads, cakes, salads and snacks
- Add mushrooms to meat dishes
- Try mushrooms on toast, in soup, in pizzas
- Eat tinned oily fish regularly
- Add peanuts to nut roasts and vegesausage mix
- Use ground almonds to thicken sauce
- Eat wholegrain bread made with yeast
- Eat brown rice instead of white
- Have a nice cup of tea!

Food for heart and blood circulation

Vitamin C, bioflavonoids and iron

These are needed to protect blood vessels and maintain healthy red blood cells. Many women have fibroids and extra-heavy periods in the peri-menopause, so iron deficiencies can be common, causing fatigue and even a feeling of depression. The main sources of vitamin C (which is usually accompanied by bioflavonoids) are dark green vegetables and citrus fruits. Many flavonoids are diuretic (promote elimination of water). Women who eat a lot of green, leafy vegetables tend to suffer less from water retention and high blood pressure.

Spirulina, kelp, nettles, watercress and parsley

These all contain iron. The last two also contain vitamin C when fresh, which increases the absorption of iron, so they are a very good iron tonic.

Plant hormones in food

There is another group of nutrients which has been receiving a great deal of attention recently. These are called **phytosterols** (plant hormones), which includes phyto-oestrogens. They are found not only in medicinal herbs but also in common foods.

How do plant hormones work?

Some plant hormones are similar in structure to human hormones, so can act in the same way. Willow, hops, dates, pomegranate, green beans and liquorice all have phytosterols, some oestrogenic, some adrenergic.

Some plants contain chemicals which can be converted into hormones in the body. Some of these are called **isoflavones**, which have become popular in supplement pills. Both these and **coumestans**, another group of hormonal precursors, are found in legumes – alfalfa, peas, clover, beans, lentils, soya and liquorice. Some herbs, such as False Unicorn Root and Wild Yam, contain diosgenin, a direct source of oestradiol (a human hormone) in commerce.

There is a whole group of herbs and spices which can be used in foods and drinks and which contain small amounts of oestrogenic compounds. This group includes Aniseed, Fennel, Fenugreek, Sarsasparilla and Sage.

The benefits of vegetable oils

Plant oils also provide building blocks for human hormones, but they have another important role in making the walls of secretory cells (such as in the ovary or uterus) work properly. All body cell walls have essential fatty acids in their structure. Animal fats can't be used for this purpose. Cell walls have to remain intact when required (to protect against leaky blood vessels) but also allow chemicals such as hormones in and out. Most women benefit from favouring plant oils over animal fats in their diet, as they help to reduce sticky cholesterol deposits in the blood vessels. You could aim at the equivalent of a teaspoon (minimum) of sunflower, olive or other seed oil per day. 'Wild' meats such as grouse, boar and goat contain more of the essential fatty acids than factory farmed meats such as beef, chicken and pork.

Recipes

All the ingredients mentioned above form the basis of the many so-called HRT cakes which have been featured in newspapers recently. Here's one I wrote earlier!

Happy hormone cake

8oz wholemeal flour
4oz chopped, dried pears
2 teaspoons baking powder
4oz sunflower seeds
1 teaspoon aniseed
1 teaspoon of fennel
1oz soya flour
6oz caster sugar
1oz flaked almonds
6oz vegetable margarine
8oz chopped dates

Vegans should add 3 tablespoons of liquid (apple juice or vegetable milk) instead of the eggs. This works perfectly!

Method

Beat the sugar and margarine together until white and fluffy. Add the beaten egg or liquid a spoonful at a time, beating well. Sift the flours, baking powder and spices, fold in lightly, add fruits and seeds.

Sprinkle flaked almonds on top. Bake in the middle of the oven on regulo 3, 160-180°C or 325-350°F, for two hours. You can vary the fruits and spices if you wish. This cake is rich in isoflavines which help you to make your own hormones.

Happy hormone breakfast

Fill a jar with:

- Flaked almonds
- Sesame seeds
- Sunflower seeds
- Chopped dates
- Dried fruits (optional)

Add this mix in generous amounts to any breakfast cereal you like, top with soya milk.

What's wrong with slimming?

It appears that there is a connection between the amount of fat women have on their body and their level of female hormones. It seems that oestrogens are stored and metabolised in fatty tissues, and that thin women are more highly represented in surveys of osteoporosis sufferers. Until there is more defining research, it may be wise to say that a little extra weight in middle age is not a bad thing. Hooray!

✨ 8 ✨

Case histories

Case 1 Joint pain and irritable bowel

Mrs B, aged 48, was diagnosed at 38 with early
menopause. She suffered from nausea, PMT, heavy
periods, irritability and bloating. She was prescribed
progesterone for three years, which was successful, but she
had to stop taking it because of suspected liver damage.
Her symptoms returned and three years ago she began
also having severe nights sweats and palpitations, which
had been intruding into the day for the previous three
months. Mrs B also complained of aching joints since her
20s, insomnia since the sweats started, alternating
diarrhoea and constipation with frequent and urgent
desire to pass water. She was advised to seek further
internal examination for fibroids, which may have caused
many of the symptoms in the pelvic area. Her priorities
were to relieve hot flushes, indigestion and aching joints.

The herbal prescription

Chasteberry – hormonal agent
Wormwood – digestive tonic
Sage – hormonal agent, astringent, antibiotic
Valerian – relaxant

Black cohosh – circulatory tonic, anti-inflammatory, hormonal agent.

Result

After two months Mrs B's digestive problems disappeared, night sweats were not as severe, the palpitations were gone and she had more energy. Her pains were also greatly reduced.

Case 2 Early menopause and disability

Miss D, aged 35, had a diagnosis from her doctor of early menopause. She suffered from cold hands and feet, sweating at night, hot flushes, breathlessness and weight gain. All her symptoms started after a serious car accident which left her badly injured and disabled, walking with crutches and in pain with very swollen knees. Lots of operations on her legs were planned to improve her condition. Miss D also had fibroids, heavy periods which were also more frequent since her accident, a constant vaginal discharge, frequent loose bowel motions, headaches, asthma and no sense of taste or smell. We agreed that many of her symptoms could be caused by stress and tension resulting from her accident and injuries. Her priority was to relieve palpitations, flushes and heavy periods.

The herbal prescription

Beth root – uterine astringent
Geranium – digestive astringent
Chasteberry – hormonal agent
Skullcap – nervine relaxant
Celery seed – relaxing anti-inflammatory, pain reliever.

Result

After two months her hot flushes were not noticeable –
only one in two weeks – she had a period of medium
flow, her knees were less swollen and she hadn't needed
to use the Ventolin inhaler. She was having two bowel
motions a day, and her sense of taste and smell was back
to normal. Blood tests at the doctor's revealed normal
hormone levels.

Case 3   Dry, blotchy skin and allergic asthma

Mrs E, aged 53, had started the menopause six months
before and had one day's light bleeding in that time. She
was suffering from hot flushes, but the main problem was
blotchy, itchy skin. Mrs E also suffered from varicose veins
and allergic asthma, and said she used to regularly drink
too much alcohol. She was advised to consider allergy
testing and elimination of dietary items one by one as
well as to increase intake of vitamin B rich foods and
plant oils. She had already resolved to cease drinking

alcohol for the time being. Her priority was to relieve hot flushes and itchy skin.

The herbal prescription

Dandelion – liver and digestive tonic
Wormwood – liver and digestive tonic
Motherwort – hormonal agent, relaxant
Sage – hormonal agent.

Result

After one month there was a great improvement, all symptoms had disappeared. Mrs E was also currently eliminating oranges and cheese from her diet to see if they were connected with the skin blotchiness and asthma. This proved to be inconclusive but her skin continued to improve on herbal medicine and we planned to treat the asthma at a later date.

Case 4   Breast cancer, Tamoxifen and night sweats

Mrs H, aged 47, had breast cancer two years before, resulting in the removal of one breast and lymph nodes. She was receiving Tamoxifen treatment. Eighteen years before one ovary had been removed because it caused severe pain. She had also undergone a hysterectomy four years after this because of very heavy periods. Mrs H was now suffering hot flushes, flu-like aches and night sweats.

She also suffered from bladder weakness since the birth of her last child and an enlarged bowel with very slow movements every two to three days. She used to take a lot of laxatives. She complained of feeling cold all the time and was currently taking Provera. Her priority was to reduce hot flushes and aches.

The first herbal prescription

Yarrow – digestive and circulatory tonic
Hawthorn – heart and circulatory tonic
Bugleweed – thyroid sedative
Horsetail – urinary system tonic.

The second herbal prescription

Yarrow – digestive and circulatory tonic
Hawthorn – herat and circulatory tonic
Boneset – for flu-type aches
Valerian – relaxant
Chasteberry – hormonal agent.

Result

The first prescription produced some improvement in all symptoms. We were careful to avoid direct oestrogenics because of worries that they might interfere with her medication. Mrs H then stopped taking Provera after discussion with her doctor, and began a second remedy. This produced a huge improvement in sleep, hot flushes were shorter and not as intense. We agreed that this probably showed that even under the influence of a chemotherapeutic agent noted for inducing hot flushes (Tamoxifen), anxiety makes them worse.

Case 5 Heavy periods, depression and anxiety

Mrs V, Aged 46, suffered from very heavy periods. She had been hospitalised for haemorrhagic bleeding on two occasions and fibroids were diagnosed at her last internal examination. She also had very tender breasts and rapidly thinning hair. Benign lumps had been removed one year before and her husband had been made redundant without warning in the same year. Her young son was suffering severe asthma attacks, with frequent hospitalisations. She had been taking anti-depressants (Diothiapin) since then. Mrs V also suffered from cyclical water retention and headaches. Her priority was to relieve heavy periods.

The herbal prescription

Shepherd's purse – uterine astringent
White deadnettle – hormonal agent
Chamomile – relaxant, anti-allergenic
Pellitory – diuretic.

Result

Mrs V's next few periods were light to normal. One year later a very small fibroid was found on examination. She was considering stopping Dothiapin and starting St John's Wort which she undertook the following year.

Case 6 Stress, water retention and fatigue

Mrs W, aged 45, as suffering from water retention, PMT, fatigue, sore breasts, dry skin and more frequent, lighter periods and a constant vaginal discharge. She was under great pressure to achieve targets in her job, was divorced three years ago and had two young children. Her priority was to relieve PMT.

The herbal prescription

Chasteberry – hormonal agent
Dandelion root – liver tonic
Dandelion leaf – diuretic
False unicorn root – hormonal agent
Kelp – metabolic alterative
Liquorice – adrenal tonic.

Result

PMT symptoms disappeared, Mrs W had more energy, and more regular, looser bowel motions. She also felt her skin was in better condition.

Case 7   Fatigue, indigestion and hot flushes

Mrs P, Aged 56, complained of fatigue, wind, constipation and catarrh. She had previously been taking HRT for mood swings, and since she stopped it had hot flushes and night sweats. Her last very light period was four months before. We decided to prioritise the digestive and hormonal dysfunction and treat the catarrh at another time, but recommended increasing plant oils and vitamin C to ensure mucus membrane health.

The herbal prescription

Lemon balm – relaxant, digestive tonic
Hops – digestive liver tonic
Aniseed – carminative
Peppermint – carminative
Chamomile – relaxant
Wild yam – oestrogenic.

Result

Great improvement in all symptoms, bowels more regular in movement, wind disappeared, night sweats and flushes moderate to unnoticeable.

Sources and resources

Nutrition – further reading

MAFF Manual of Nutrition (HMSO). A brief guide to the contents of major foods and dietary guidelines with daily requirements. This book was used by every home economics student and teacher from the 1950s until the 1980s when cookery and nutrition became design and labelling!

Identifying herbs – further reading

The Concise British Flora W. Keble-Martin (Ebury Press). The author was a vicar who spent all his spare time painting wild flowers. This is a remarkable book which captures the essence of each flower and plant. Better than photos for identifying difficult to recognise subjects. Not easy to use, as the plants are arranged in families, but worth persevering.

Exercise

The British Wheel of Yoga, 25 Jermyn Street, Sleaford, Lincolnshire NG34 7RU. Tel: (01529) 303233. The main association for yoga teachers and those interested in yoga. Hatha yoga is the type which has most general application – it is yoga for health. This is mainly what you will find being taught in evening classes and lunchtime sessions. It consists of a series of tone and stretch exercises which

have been developed over thousands of years in India.
Most teachers include some exercises from other strands
of yoga as these are more directly designed to relax the
mind and are associated with meditation. Some people
with strong religious faiths are afraid that yoga involves
taking up a mystic religion. This isn't true – the
meditations are designed to make you aware of your mind
and enable you to empty it. They can be performed by
members of any religious group.

Seeds

King's Seeds, Monk's Farm, Coggeshall Road, Kelvedon,
Essex CO5 9PG. Tel (01376) 572456. The only company
in Britain selling a wide variety of wild flower and herb
seeds. Previously Suffolk Herbs, it has recently been taken
over.

Samuel Dobie and Son, Long Rd, Paignton, Devon TQ4
7SX. Tel (01803) 696444. Dobie's Seeds sells a wide range
of flower and vegetable seeds, with a good selection of
culinary herbs.

Seeing herbs

The Chelsea Physic Garden, Royal Hospital Walk (entrance
in Cheyne Walk), London (Sloane Square tube). Tel:
(0207) 352 5646. Probably the best collection in Britain,
begun in the 17th century, brilliant teas and cakes,
exquisite pleasure to walk round. Open Sundays from

2pm and some weekdays. Run by volunteers (who make the cakes!).

Buying dried herbs and preparations

Alban Mills Herbs, 38 Sandridge Road, St Albans AL1 4AS. Tel (01727) 858243. *www.lsgmillscare4free.net*. A very large range of medicinal and culinary herbs and spices, creams, oils, syrups, tablets, toiletries and essential oils. Small amounts no problem.

Gardening

The Henry Doubleday Research Association, Ryton in Dunsmore, near Coventry, Warwickshire. The Association has its own seed catalogue, run by Chase organics, and a magazine for subscribers which gives advice on organic gardening and news of organic projects in Britain and abroad.

Gardener's Question Time (2pm Sunday Radio 4, repeated in the day-time during the week) has been offering gardening advice from a panel of experts to live audiences for generations. *Gardener's World* (8.30 BBC2) still offers a designer-free zone of real gardening.

Consulting herbalists

The National Institute of Medical Herbalists (NIMH), 56 Longbrook Street, Exeter, Devon EX46AH. Tel: (01392) 426022. *www.btinternet.com/~nimh/*. Established in 1864 to promote training and standards in herbal medicine. It is the oldest body of professional herbalists in the world. Members train for four years to a BSc in Herbal Medicine, which involves herbal pharmacology, medical sciences and pharmacognosy (the science of recognising herbal compounds and materials).

Representatives of the NIMH sit on government committees and are involved in decisions on the safety of herbal medicines in Britain and Europe.

Counselling and talking therapies

Self-help books are abundant. You will need to read more than one to get an idea of the different sorts of talking therapies.

Patient support groups

These are extremely useful for sharing problems and solutions. Ask in your local library for the *Directory of Associations* which contains all national associations and is updated annually. The current secretarial address of the Menopause support groups are there.

List of herbs within their applications

Hormonal agents

Anemone
Beth root
Black cohosh
Chasteberry
False unicorn root
Hops
Motherwort
Nettle
Raspberry leaf
Red clover
Sage
Shepherd's purse
Squaw vine
White deadnettle
Wild yam

Circulatory tonics

Buckwheat
Ginkgo
Hawthorn
Horsechestnut
Motherwort
Passionflower
Rue

Iron tonics

Couch grass
Nettles
Parsley
Water cress
Yellow dock

Relaxants

Black cohosh
Chamomile
Cowslips
Cramp bark
Kava-kava
Lemon Balm
Limeflowers
Passionflower
Skullcap
St John's wort
Valerian
Vervein
Wild yam

Digestive Tonics

Agrimony
Chamomile
Gentian
Rosemary
Sage
Thyme
Wormwood

General index